# YOGA
## THE GREATER TRADITION

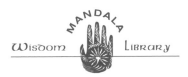

Wisdom MANDALA Library

**MANDALA**
PUBLISHING

PO Box 3088
San Rafael, CA 94912
www.mandalapublishing.com

Library of Congress Cataloging-in-Publication Data available.

ISBN: 978-1-60109-016-4

REPLANTED PAPER

Insight Editions, in association with Roots of Peace, will plant
two trees for each tree used in the manufacturing of this book.
Roots of Peace is an internationally renowned humanitarian
organization dedicated to eradicating land mines worldwide and
converting war-torn lands into productive farms and wildlife
habitats. Together, we will plant two million fruit and nut trees in
Afghanistan and provide farmers there with the skills and support
necessary for sustainable land use.

Manufactured in China by Insight Editions
www.insighteditions.com

10 9 8 7 6 5 4 3 2

The content of this book is provided for informational purposes
only and is not intended to diagnose, treat, or cure any
conditions without the assistance of a trained practitioner. If
you are experiencing any medical condition, seek care from an
appropriate licensed professional.

# YOGA

## THE GREATER TRADITION

### DAVID FRAWLEY

MANDALA
PUBLISHING

San Rafael, California

# TABLE

*Preface*......**7**

*Part 1: Yoga and Its Greater Teachings*......**9**
What Is Yoga?......**10**
The Greater Yoga Tradition......**17**
The Profound Philosophy of Yoga......**27**
The Vast Literature of Yoga......**35**

*Part 2: The Greater Practices of Yoga*......**47**
The Integral System of Classical Yoga......**48**
YAMAS & NIYAMAS: Yogic Values and Lifestyle......**53**
ASANA: The Yogic Stilling of the Physical Body......**58**
PRANAYAMA: Developing the Power of the Breath......**62**
PRATYAHARA: The Yogic Internalization of the Senses......**67**
The Inner Yoga of Meditation......**72**

# OF CONTENTS

JNANA YOGA: The Path of Knowledge......79

BHAKTI YOGA: The Path of Devotion......82

Tantric and Energy Yogas......85

Yoga as Mantra and Chanting......89

Yoga Therapy, Ayurveda, and Healing......95

Conclusion:
Entering the Universe of Yoga......102

Appendix and Resources......105

Glossary of Terms......106

End Notes......107

About the Author......111

Colophon......112

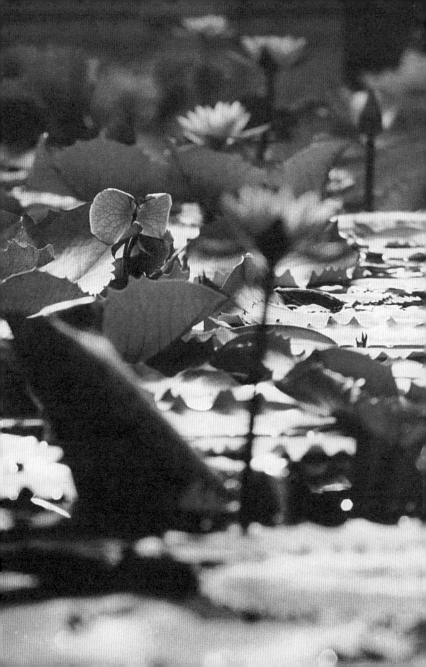

# Preface ✣

As yoga continues to grow in popularity as a modern exercise and fitness movement, it is important to notice the greater spiritual tradition that forms its core. Besides an elaborate system of body postures, or asanas, yoga contains an entire philosophy and way of life that addresses the purpose of our existence and our higher potential, both individually and as a species.

This slim volume intends to shed light on the greater tradition and teachings of yoga, which provide an integral approach that can harmonize our individual and collective existence. My aim is to provide yoga students with a new vision of the universe of yoga in all its vastness. Addressing the greater tradition of yoga in a few pages is no easy task, but I hope to provide some keys to take students forward on their journeys.

This book may lead you to other publications on yoga and its related traditions of Ayurveda, Vedic astrology, Tantra and Vedanta. I hope it will encourage a deeper study of yoga, as well as of its vast literature and many methods and levels of practice.

David Frawley
Santa Fe, New Mexico

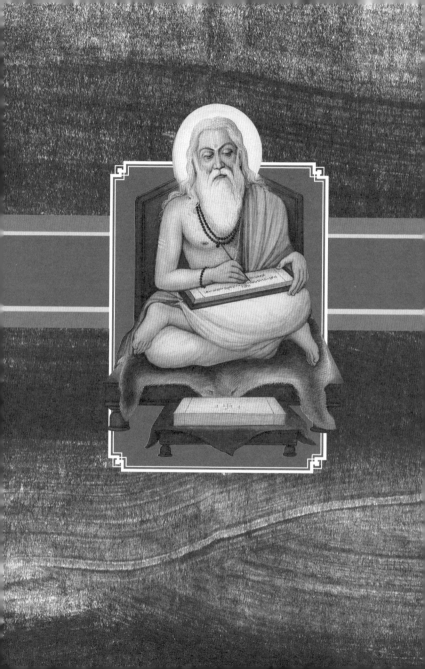

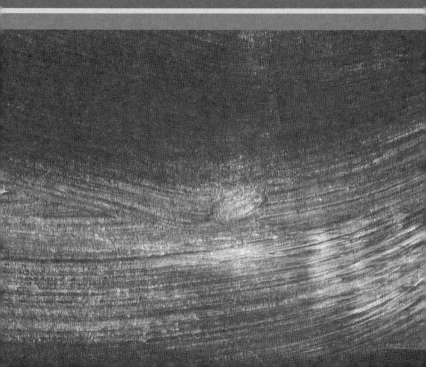

PART ONE

# Yoga and Its Greater Teachings

# What Is

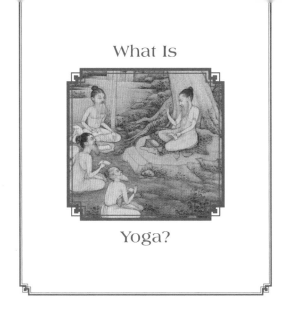

## Yoga?

Like many people, you may have taken some yoga classes and perhaps mastered a few yoga postures. Still, you may not be aware of everything yoga has to offer, not only for the body but also for the mind and our deeper consciousness and higher awareness. What is yoga really about, in its entire depth and breadth?

Today we are familiar with the popular media image of yoga as an exercise system that affords its followers flexible, beautiful, and slim figures. Such yoga bodies abound on the covers of health magazines throughout the world. Yoga exercise classes are found in almost every community around the globe and have become popular with rich and famous athletes and celebrities. This trendy, commercialized version of yoga blends well with the pursuit of fitness, affluence, and personal happiness that dominates modern culture. We are told that if we practice yoga regularly, we will lose weight, look better, have more supple bodies, and handle stress better.

Although all of these things are possible, yoga possesses an additional spiritual mystique of a different order. Traditional yoga reflects an entire set of consciousness-raising practices that include chanting mantras and practicing various forms of meditation. It is not concerned as much with physical or personal well-being as with spiritual development. Alongside the yoga body are the aura of a yogic mind, a yogic consciousness, and a higher yogic state of bliss or self-realization beyond time and space.

This deeper mystical yoga has its own particular fascination and magic. It draws our attention to gurus, ashrams, and India, the homeland of yoga, with its exotic temples and vast tropical landscape. It brings to mind the image of mysterious yogis with supernatural powers who, having conquered death and sorrow, live high in the Himalayas.

Although not altogether absent in modern yoga movements, this spiritual landscape of yoga is not always apparent to the average yoga student. It also figures in popular yoga books such as *Autobiography of a Yogi* by Paramahansa Yogananda, one of the first yogis who, in the twentieth century, brought yoga to the West. The early yoga movements that spread outside of India were actually more of this spiritual type, in which exercises of postures and breath control do not play such an important role.

So what is yoga all about? Are we really getting the best possible benefit from yoga through a good workout in a yoga class? Or are we just skimming the surface of the ocean of yoga that can take us into a totally different dimension of awareness?

This book is designed to introduce the reader to the greater universe of yoga, the yoga of higher consciousness.

It explains yoga as a comprehensive sacred science of body, mind, and spirit, designed to put us in harmony with all of existence. While yoga certainly includes physical health and well-being, it extends far beyond these to true happiness and everlasting bliss. Yoga is a spiritual quest to know the inner reality of the universe, the divine, God, the absolute, or whatever one may wish to call the highest truth.

## Defining Yoga ✿

A good place to start our examination of yoga is to look at how yoga has been defined over the centuries. Yoga derives from the Sanskrit root *yuj*, meaning "work," "coordination," and "integration." Yoga is connected to the English term *yoke*, as in yoking a horse to a chariot. Specifically yoga is defined as "union," a state of oneness with the divine as our own inmost self. In this sense, yoga is the integration of our individual being with the greater cosmic reality. It is a means of reunification with the higher awareness that is our true origin, goal, and deepest nature.

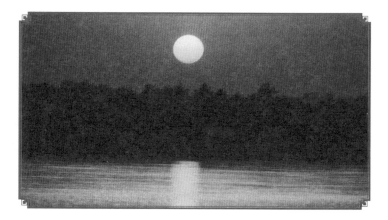

Yoga has also generally referred to various spiritual practices used in India since time immemorial. Such practices not only include asana but also ritual, pranayama, mantra, chanting, contemplation, and meditation—all the various tools for developing higher consciousness.

So there are five primary yoga paths:

1. **Jnana Yoga** *(the yoga of knowledge):*
   self-realization through inner knowledge and insight

2. **Bhakti Yoga** *(the yoga of devotion):*
   self-realization through devotion or divine love

3. **Karma Yoga** *(the yoga of service):*
   self-realization through selfless work and sacred ritual

4. **Raja Yoga** *(the royal yoga):*
   self-realization through a combination of knowledge, devotion, and work

5. **Hatha Yoga** *(the yoga of technique):*
   self-realization through a combination of asana, pranayama, mantra, and meditation practices

While these five are primary, the number of possible yoga paths is unlimited. Many types of yoga have long existed in the numerous traditions of ancient, medieval, and modern India. Every major spiritual, religious, and cultural group in the Indian tradition (whether Hindu, Buddhist, or Jain) includes some form of yoga in its practices, principles, or aspirations.

These Indian yoga practices have parallels in mystical traditions throughout the world, going back to the time of ancient Egypt, if not before. Yet these inner teachings appear best preserved in the yoga tradition, developed and integrated into a harmonious whole, more so perhaps than any other tradition. This is probably because as a culture India has always honored individual spiritual experience over any outer authority, dogma, belief, or institution. The continuity of its inner teachings has never been broken since the earliest era.

Today many people speak of the types of yoga they have encountered, such as Iyengar, Astanga, or Kundalini. However, by this they usually mean different styles of asana practice, or yoga postures, rather than the broader spiritual paths mentioned above. Most of these asana styles are recent inventions, although some are based on ancient principles. To understand the essence of yoga, it is important to look at yoga as a comprehensive spiritual path, not just as a variety of asana methods.

Modern asana yoga is often called *Hatha Yoga*. Yet traditional Hatha Yoga does not consist primarily of asana practice (which it does cover in some detail) but directs greater attention to pranayama and meditation, the use of energetic techniques to develop higher awareness.

Among the many definitions of yoga in the traditional literature, an important one is given in the Yoga Sutras, the prime text of Raja Yoga, attributed to the sage Patanjali. The Yoga Sutras define yoga as *citta vritti nirodha*, which translates as "calming the modifications of the mind." This definition of yoga is primarily a definition of meditation, which is the central focus of traditional yoga teachings and allows the student to abide in his or her higher self.[1]

Other common ancient definitions of yoga include "the state of balance,"[2] "skill in action,"[3] "release from the causes of suffering,"[4] "steady concentration of the senses,"[5] "the beginning and end of practice,"[6] and so on. Many of these definitions come from the Bhagavad Gita, which addresses the subject of yoga from many angles. Other ancient definitions of yoga come from the Upanishads, which mainly refer to yoga as the "yoga of meditation"[7] and the "yoga of the inner self."[8] Both texts are older than the Yoga Sutras and are accepted as authoritative sources.

It is important to note that none of these classical definitions refers to yoga as asana, exercise, or even as a healing therapy.[9] This is because traditionally yoga is a spiritual practice, called *sadhana* in Sanskrit, followed by those who are not satisfied with the beliefs and rituals of outer religious activity. Yoga sadhana aims to establish direct contact with the divine or higher consciousness. Yoga as a form of exercise or therapy has existed alongside, but secondary to, the primary pursuit of union with ultimate reality.

From the standpoint of those who pursue yoga as a sadhana, particularly the yogas of devotion or knowledge, asana may not have much importance. The exceptions are the paths emphasizing yoga techniques such as Hatha Yoga and sometimes Raja Yoga, which propagate special asanas as part of pranayama and meditation approaches.

## Yoga, Self-Realization, and the Divine ✖

Traditionally, yoga aims toward self-realization, a term most of us can relate to. We all want to realize our higher potential, to be or gain all that we can in life. Terms such as *self-empowerment, self-esteem,* and *self-promotion* abound in today's popular literature. However, yoga is not concerned with the realization of our human ego or outer self, our personal talents, desires, or ambitions. The yogic self is our inner being, the higher consciousness within us that is linked to the universe as a whole. Yogic self-realization concerns reaching an awareness beyond time and space, rather than any type of temporary material fulfillment. It is designed to take us to the self within us, which is part and parcel of the divine.

Yoga is also said to be a path to *god-realization*, a term some of us may have a harder time relating to. If we believe in God, we may doubt that any human being can become one with God. If we don't believe in God, we may regard yoga as another religious illusion. So we must note that yoga looks at the divine very differently than we normally do. Yoga regards God, or the divine, as a power of consciousness that exists inside us and simultaneously pervades the entire universe. This view of the divine as pure consciousness has affinities not only with religion but also with science, art, and mysticism. It is not about belief but about experiencing the true nature of reality, which is universal.

Yoga is a tradition that helps us achieve our ultimate well-being, not only physical but also psychological and spiritual. For this purpose, it employs an entire array of practices relative to body, mind, heart, and inner awareness. The rich and complex asana tradition that we see in modern yoga has its counterparts in profound and detailed yoga systems of pranayama, mantra, and meditation. Once we understand the greater scope of yoga, we open ourselves to the possibility of connecting with an unbounded realm of consciousness and bliss.

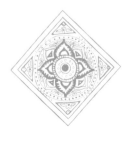

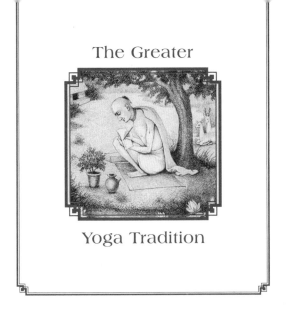

# The Greater

# Yoga Tradition

In the broad sense of the term, yoga is a vast tradition extending from ancient history, covering numerous teachers, teachings, groups, and practices in India, nearby regions, and beyond. To understand yoga in its deeper sense, we have to explore the vastness of the greater yoga tradition.

## Patanjali and the Yoga Sutras

A good place to start the study of the yoga tradition is through an ancient book called the Yoga Sutras, compiled by the sage Patanjali, who is said to have lived over two thousand years ago. Some people call the Yoga Sutras the textbook or even the Bible of yoga. Though it is not the only, the most detailed, or even the oldest yogic text, the Yoga Sutras remains an important compilation of yoga principles and practices. Patanjali reflected the main yoga teachings of his day as well as older yoga traditions. His short aphorisms have remained an authoritative summary of yoga teachings down to the present day.

The first thing one notices when studying the Yoga Sutras is that its teachings are short and cryptic. Sutras are a branch of Sanskrit literature that summarizes major points, a kind of shorthand. They are not detailed books but resemble a list of topics or chapter headings requiring special commentaries to make sense of them. The Yoga Sutras also contains many technical Sanskrit terms that have no English equivalents. These include terms for higher states of consciousness[10] that our science seems to know little about.

There are numerous books, both traditional and modern, that serve as commentaries on the Yoga Sutras. Traditional commentaries (such as the famous ancient Vyasa commentary) were written for an informed Indian audience centuries ago. They are as difficult to understand as the Sutras themselves and introduce additional Sanskrit terms.

Among the more accessible modern commentaries are academic studies of the Yoga Sutras by scholars who have never practiced yoga and may not even value it. There are also versions of the Sutras by modern yoga teachers who may not know Sanskrit but rely on other, possibly inaccurate translations. Comparing modern commentaries shows that the same Sutra can be interpreted in very different ways.

However, one thing is clear after any real examination of the Yoga Sutras: traditional yoga does not afford much importance to asanas, or yoga postures. Of the more than two hundred Sutras in the Yoga Sutras, only two address the topic of asana. Though asanas are the main aspect of modern yoga, from the small amount of attention given them in the Yoga Sutras, they seem to be the least significant part of classical yoga.

If we look at the traditional literature on yoga, we see that the exercise-based approach to yoga that is popular today is, at best, one aspect of a many-sided yoga tradition and, at worst, not representative of it at all. A quick glance at the yoga tradition will reveal that it is much more than what we have likely considered it.

If we examine other traditional texts on yoga, we discover that Patanjali is just one of many ancient yoga teachers. Yoga and its related terminology are found in numerous books from India, reflecting a variety of traditions and referencing many different groups, most of which do not mention Patanjali at all. No single teacher or text dominates the yoga tradition.

We cannot stereotype yoga as one particular practice, such as asana, or as the teaching of any one group or person. Yoga is about the maximum integration of all aspects of our nature and can be studied from many angles. The essence of yoga resides in its ability to harmonize all the diverse factors of our experience. While this view of yoga may seem confusing at first, it allows us to take a new journey into the universe of yoga and look at life in an integral way.

## Is Yoga a Religion? ❧

When people begin to look beyond asanas, one of the first concerns they have with yoga is whether or not it is a religion. Will taking up the deeper practices of yoga require adopting a particular religious belief? Will it require that we give up our current religion? Some of us may not want to follow any religion at all. Does one have to believe in God to practice yoga?

Any real examination of the yoga tradition soon shows us that yoga has an undeniable religious and spiritual side. Traditional yoga is concerned with the divine, our inner being, and the achievement of immortality, though it may define these concepts differently than does Western religious thought.

The yoga traditions of India contain monastic orders, temples, and holy places. They have special rituals and congregations, including massive religious festivals such as the famous Kumbha Melas, where tens of millions of people come together at sacred rivers to visit with great yogis and sages from throughout the country. Yoga has its own venerable history of saints, sages, and seers extending long before the currently known religions emerged. Yogic ascetics and hermits, the famous sadhus of India, can still be found in large numbers in the Himalayas, with their special dress, vows, and austerities. Those who have renounced the world commonly use the yoga practices found in the Yoga Sutras.

One can find very little in the religions of the world that is not present in yoga, regarding both practices and philosophies. Yogic teachings contain views that resemble theism, emphasizing a single creator of the universe, worshipped as father and mother, friend, beloved, and master. Other yogic teachings resemble polytheism, honoring many different deities and recognizing a divine face in every hill and brook, much like pantheism or nature worship. Other yoga teachings are monistic, emphasizing one reality or absolute called *Brahman*, which means "beyond even God, the soul, and the universe." Many yoga teachings combine and reconcile such seemingly contradictory views into a greater harmony, finding a place for each.

The yoga tradition resembles a collection of religions under the banner of yoga as a set of spiritual practices. In this way it seems that yoga can accommodate any number of religious views as long as they aim at the goal of inner realization. We must remember that the original meaning of the term *religion*, "to link together," is similar to that of *yoga* as "union and integration."

How does yoga relate to the Hindu and Vedic traditions, in the context of which classical yoga arises? If we look at Indian culture, we find that some aspect of yoga is integral to the entire Hindu way of life, permeating Indian music, dance, martial arts, medicine, poetry, and philosophy. In ancient India all ways of knowledge could be paths of yoga, even such studies as grammar or astronomy. Because the Vedic tradition is not only the oldest but also the most diverse and complex of the world's religious traditions, yoga's connection with it infuses a similar vastness and many-sidedness to its scope. Yoga includes religion, art, science, and culture as part of an inner orientation to know one's true nature. It is a sacred way of life that helps all that we do, which is what real religion is all about to begin with.

## Yoga and Experiential Spirituality

Though most aspects of religion have counterparts in yoga, yoga is more individually than institutionally based and cannot be reduced to a single religious system or orientation. Yoga emphasizes spiritual practice of a personal nature. It enables us to develop a direct experience of the higher truth within our own minds and hearts, and it is not satisfied with mere belief as enough for our inner welfare.

This does not mean that we can practice yoga any way we want and still do it justice. To truly practice yoga requires dedication, commitment, and discipline, including a willingness to question everything about ourselves, our values, and even our identity. In the inner sense yoga is an unrelenting pursuit of the truth of who we are and what the universe really is all about.

Though not resting on one religious belief, this deeper, or inner, yoga requires that we have a spiritual orientation in life and be receptive to the higher consciousness behind the universe. It leads us to a deeper understanding of our true being, not only beyond religious barriers but also beyond all time and space. Yoga can perhaps be best described as a form of experiential spirituality, using universal principles applied at an individual level. In this way yoga can reconcile both the religious and nonreligious sides of our nature.

Yoga is usually based on personal study with a teacher, who is linked to a lineage or tradition of yoga with its own specific guidelines. There are many different groups in the greater tradition of yoga. Each of these movements has its particular requirements that must be honored if we wish to join them, which may not always be easy. Some yoga groups may be more devotional or more ascetic than others.

Yoga turns religion and spirituality into a set of resources, attempting to offer a wide variety to everyone. Yoga encourages you to "take the path that most directly leads you to experience the inner truth of your own nature." Yoga is a universal teaching, conveying that the entire universe dwells within us. The entire universe—all time, space, and existence—dwells in the small space within our hearts. Becoming *that* is yoga.

# The Science of Yoga 🪷

Yoga is a way of knowledge, a science. Yoga proceeds systematically to study, explore, and unlock the various powers, faculties, and levels of awareness within us.

Yet yoga is not an outer science such as physics, which can be reduced to mathematical formulas, or an analytical science such as psychology, which can be examined at a personal level. Yoga is an inner science of experience in consciousness. We perform its experiments on ourselves, on our own bodies and minds. Its results are not simply physical or quantitative but qualitative, providing a new way of experiencing life and perceiving reality.

Yoga is a sacred science. It requires that we approach life reverently. It is about understanding the essence of things, not merely taking apart or analyzing their outer forms. In this way, yoga is related to other sacred sciences. Yoga has traditionally been aligned to Vedic medicine or *Ayurveda*, Vedic astrology or *Jyotish*, Vedic architecture or *Vastu,* and Vedic mathematics, all of which have a yogic orientation.

# The Yoga Tradition 🪷

What is this greater tradition of yoga? First of all, it is the continuity of yoga teachers, practices, and views that have existed throughout history. Specifically it refers to those groups who have consciously aligned themselves with yoga and developed its philosophies and practices. While this is not a rigidly defined association, it does have its identity and connections.

To understand the yoga tradition we need to know more about the background from which it arose. In this regard yoga takes us back to the concept of *dharma*, another term that is difficult to translate. Yoga teaches us that we live in a universe pervaded by intelligence and possessing a deep inner order and harmony. The laws of the greater conscious universe are called *dharma*.

Specifically yoga takes us back to *Sanatana Dharma*, the eternal dharma, which postulates an unchanging and universal truth behind all of life. Sanatana Dharma is the original name for the greater Hindu tradition, and Buddhists and Jains have used the term as well. Certain modern writers have brought up a similar concept with that of perennial philosophy, the transcendent truth behind all the religions and philosophies of the world.

The main idea behind Sanatana Dharma is that there is one universal spirituality, which takes different forms in different countries, cultures, and individuals, not only through religion but also through art, music, science, or just day-to-day living. Therefore yoga is not a tradition of name or form; it doesn't rest upon a label. It is a tradition that aims at the integration of all our faculties into a cosmic higher awareness. It includes whatever helps us to do this. We could say that yoga is the religion of nature, life, and consciousness beyond outer labels. All creatures in all worlds will discover some form of yoga in their quest for higher awareness.

The history of yoga is intertwined with the history of India and its great spiritual traditions. Every strata of India's past has its yoga or inner practices. There are figures seated in meditation poses and performing yoga asanas found in the ancient seals over five thousand years old, from the ancient cities of India.[11] India's greatest epic story, the over two-thousand-year-old Mahabharata, is filled with yogic teachings and practices.

Yoga was a common practice among the great leaders who brought about the independence of India in modern times, such as Mahatma Gandhi, Rabindranath Tagore, and Sri Aurobindo. In fact, the modern revival of yoga in India was an important part of India's reawakening as a nation and culture. We find a continuous flow of teachers, teachings, images, and artifacts testifying to this great tradition of yoga and its unbroken continuity over time. While the details of these yoga teachings may change over time, their essence remains.

Yoga also has had historical influences outside of India as well as connections with many spiritual movements the world over. These connections can be harder to trace, and it is difficult to ascertain whether they derive from a direct contact or a common discovery. But the current global popularity of yoga probably is not happening for the first time!

## Modern Yoga ✺

Over time, modern yoga has become a movement of its own, related to, but often different from, classical yoga. Yoga was introduced to the Western world by a disciple of Paramahansa Ramakrishna, Swami Vivekananda, who first visited the United States in 1893. The first major yoga guru to set up residence in the United States was Paramahansa Yogananda, who settled in the United States in 1920. Starting in the 1960s, many yoga gurus came to America and spread the teachings of yoga in different forms. Such teachers and their disciples brought the teachings of yoga to the other countries of the world as well.

For these early yoga movements, yoga was mainly a spiritual practice allied to meditation, mantra, and devotion. Yet asana as the physical aspect of yoga appealed to the outer-minded Western audience. So, over time asana became the visible face of yoga, particularly with yoga teachers sitting in the lotus pose! Asana became a vehicle for introducing people to yoga, starting with its most accessible aspect, the physical body.

Then, in the 1970s, asana came to dominate the yoga scene through a new set of yoga teachers from India that aimed at precision asana practice as the most important aspect of yoga. Today this asana view of yoga is so prevalent that many people have forgotten the older, deeper, and more extensive spiritual side of yoga. Today you can find many very good asana teachers in the West and much innovation in their practices. Yet only a few of these teachers may really understand the spiritual dimension of yoga.

While modern yoga reflects aspects of the yoga tradition, it is important to realize that the tradition contains more than what we find in the yoga popular today. Even great yoga masters who have taught in the West have not always been able to impart their fullest or deepest teachings. We are just beginning to discover the universe of yoga, though we may have made some progress.

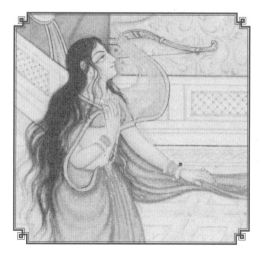

# The Profound

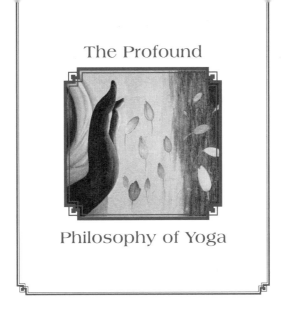

## Philosophy of Yoga

Yoga is based upon a profound philosophy of life and consciousness. It is not a system of mere practices devoid of any theoretical background. The philosophy of yoga is one of the greatest in the world and can be the subject for a lifetime of study and contemplation.

To practice yoga at a deeper level, it is necessary to have a yogic view of life. In the West we tend to be practical people who prefer a how-to approach. We may be suspicious of theories and ideologies, preferring to start practicing yoga rather than study it. However, we must remember that any science has its body of knowledge and special terminology. Performing chemistry experiments by mixing chemical compounds at will, without having a background in chemistry, may cause an explosion. Similarly one needs an understanding of yoga philosophy to practice yoga effectively, without causing damage by doing it wrong. While theory without practice cannot take us far, practice without any theory also has its limitations.

When we speak of the philosophy of yoga, we are not referring to any mere intellectual, academic, or speculative discipline. Yoga philosophy shows us how to understand the world and ourselves within our own awareness. Yoga philosophy is a practical philosophy of self-observation and inner inquiry. We learn it by applying it in our daily lives.

## The Yogic Mind and Heart ❋

The purpose of yoga is to cultivate a yogic mind as the vehicle that transports us to the yogic consciousness that is one with all. The philosophy and worldview of yoga is designed to help us develop this yogic mind.

The yogic mind is a deeper intelligence that grasps the fundamental laws of life, the universal dharmas. It sees all things as sacred and part of one greater conscious being. This yogic mind is not based upon mere reason, imagination, or calculation. It reflects a higher level of intuition, insight, and inner experience—an ability to look beyond mere information to enduring principles and eternal values.

This yogic mind is called *buddhi* in Sanskrit, which is connected to the term *Buddha*, "the enlightened One." The buddhi is not simply the outer, intellectual, or rational mind. This higher mind or intelligence of yoga does have its rationality, but it is not that of the outer world or senses. It is based on the rationality that the eternal alone is real and the transient, however fascinating, ultimately is unreal. The buddhi connects us to cosmic intelligence, not simply to the inventions and opinions of the human mind.

Yoga teaches us that the origin of the mind is in the heart, much as the old European dictum, "as he thinketh in his heart, so is he." The inner mind, or buddhi, unites direct knowing with pure feeling. It is as much a power of what we call the heart as what we call the mind. The yogic mind can be called the mind or intelligence of the inner heart. It has a quality of devotion and faith, not merely in a particular name and form, but in the divine intelligence governing the universe.

In the yogic view, the heart is the seat of the soul, the higher self, and the divine presence within us. Yet this heart is not the physical or emotional heart but the spiritual heart, called *hridaya* in Sanskrit.[12] To really practice yoga, we must develop a yogic mind and heart. The yogic mind discovers unity through inner knowledge and meditation; the yogic heart discovers unity through inner devotion and surrender.

## The Yogic View of Self ✵

The yogic pursuit of self-realization rests upon a particular understanding of the nature of the self. According to yoga philosophy, our true self is neither body nor mind but pure consciousness. This higher self or soul, called the *Atman*, is distinct from the ordinary ego. It is our inner being, the part of our nature that is unchanging and eternal. It is often defined as the "inner witness," relative to which the movements of the mind, emotions, and senses are but outer fluctuations. Yoga is a means of helping us understand our inner being and holding our awareness within it.

Our true self, or Atman, connects us to all of existence as a manifestation of the divine. It takes us beyond our bodily, intellectual, and even human views of self to a deeper oneness with the Infinite. To reach this inner self requires that we place our body consciousness in the background, go beyond the mind and experience the divine reality directly within us.

## The Yogic Worldview ✿

Yoga contains its own view of the world, the universe, humanity, civilization, and history. The yoga tradition has its own school of thought, perhaps more complex and certainly more deeply focused on the spiritual than the dominant philosophies of our present culture.

First, yoga instructs that we live in a conscious universe, known as the *Purusha* or "the Cosmic Being." The purpose of yoga is to realize the Cosmic Being, the conscious universe within us. In the yogic view, the entire universe—past, present, and future—dwells within our hearts and can be grasped as part of our deepest nature.

Second, yoga orients us to nature, which it calls *prakriti*. It tells us that to know our inner being, or Purusha, we must harmonize our outer nature, or prakriti, according to which our bodies and minds function. Yoga is closely connected to nature and teaches us that a return to natural living is the foundation for the spiritual life. But in the yogic view, nature is not some unconscious force; it is pervaded by the light of consciousness, reflecting a deeper wisdom and grace.

Yoga teaches us that there are three great qualities
called *gunas* that operate behind
all the processes of nature.

**Sattva**: *intelligence, light, harmony, balance, calm, devotion*
**Rajas**: *energy, life, movement, change, passion, agitation*
**Tamas**: *matter, inertia, stasis, darkness, dullness, resistance*

Yoga practice consists of two stages. The first is developing
sattva guna, or harmony and light, in the body and mind.
The second is going beyond sattva guna to the Purusha or
higher self that transcends the outer world of time and space.
To develop sattva guna requires that we live a life of honesty,
truthfulness, nonviolence, compassion, and devotion. To go
beyond sattva guna means that we must learn to perceive our
true self as the reality and not simply regard virtuous living as
an end in itself.

Yoga teaches us to develop sattva guna in our food,
behavior, relationships, work, and spiritual practices. It
teaches us to let go of *rajas*, or turbulence, aggression, and
agitation within us. And it helps us to remove *tamas*, the
darkness, inertia, ignorance, and confusion we might have.

## Doing Yoga or Being Yoga? ⚘

In the modern world, we are caught up in a culture of doing.
This involves traveling, working out, taking programs and
seminars, pursuing a variety of entertainments, and the many
things that have come to fill up our hectic daily lives. If we
approach yoga, we usually want to know what yoga can do for
us and what yoga practices we can add to our repertoire of
activities to make our schedule more complete.

However, real yoga is about *being* rather than simply *doing*. Yoga teaches us to know ourselves, which is not a product of outer activity. It teaches us to contact our inner being, which is obscured by outer actions and pursuits. Yoga provides us a great revelation in this regard. We don't ultimately need to do anything at all to be happy; we need only come to rest within our true nature. This resembles returning to the center of the universe, which everything else must move around!

Real yoga is about nondoing. Much of our unhappiness, and even disease, arises from the fact that we are already doing too much. We have no time, not even for ourselves, much less for our loved ones. We are constantly on the go and yet never seem to arrive at any place where we want to stay for very long.

Yoga is about doing less and being more present wherever we are and with whatever we need to do. Yoga is not simply something new but a better way of using the faculties and resources we already have. Yoga asanas are about moving the body more slowly, ultimately bringing it into stillness. Yogic meditation is about slowing down the mind and creating deep calm and unwavering inner peace that does not require any outer entertainment. A yogic lifestyle is about not bringing any harm or interference into the lives of others.

Yoga is not as much a new achievement as a means of letting go and relaxing into the infinite. Yoga philosophy is a philosophy of being. You are all that you need to be. But to discover that, you must move aside the veils of the body, mind, and senses and uncover the essence of your being.

## Yoga and the End of All Suffering

The main problem in life is suffering, regardless of where we live or what we do. Suffering comes to all of us in one form or another; to the rich and poor, the young and old alike. This sorrow may be physical, emotional, or circumstantial. It may be personal, relative to the state of our country, or to our planet as a whole. Therefore one of the most important questions we can ask ourselves is, "How can we put a permanent end to all suffering?"

Yoga addresses the issue of suffering as one of its prime philosophical considerations. Yoga was devised as the sovereign means to end all suffering. Yogic practices not only promote physical and psychological well-being, but also yoga as a whole is aimed at eliminating spiritual suffering.

Yoga philosophy specifically addresses the spiritual component of suffering. Yoga instructs that spiritual suffering is caused by confusing the seer with the seen, the self with its instruments, the eternal with the transient, the real with the unreal, and being with nonbeing. To put it simply, spiritual suffering arises from the identification of our true nature with the limitations of body and mind. If we learn to witness the conditions of body and mind, whether painful or pleasurable, and not identify them as our own, we can go beyond all suffering.

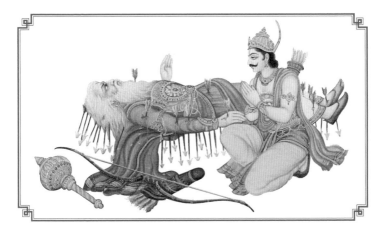

## Yoga defines spiritual suffering according to the five *kleshas*, or "factors of affliction":

1. **Avidya**: ignorance of our true nature
2. **Asmita**: egoism or false identification of our inner being with the body and mind
3. **Raga**: attraction to the factors that bring us personal happiness
4. **Dvesha**: repulsion by the factors that bring us personal pain
5. **Abhinivesha**: clinging to bodily existence

Physical suffering comes to everyone because even the healthiest person must eventually get old and die. Similarly, psychological suffering is there for everyone because life always has experiences that are not to our personal liking or preference. However, putting an end to spiritual suffering, which means no longer identifying one's true being with the body and mind, frees us from physical and psychological suffering as well. Even if outer suffering occurs, the yogi no longer sees such pain as belonging to him but witnesses it from a higher awareness. For those seeking the complete end to all suffering, yoga is the way.

Yoga is called a kind of *Moksha Dharma*. It addresses *moksha*, the "liberation of the spirit," which is regarded as the highest goal of life in Indian philosophy. We all seek freedom from pain and limitation but confuse the freedom to get or do whatever we want with real freedom. Real freedom is freedom from fear, desire, and attachment—freedom from body and mind. It is the freedom to be everything and exist forever. In this inner freedom can be found both the end of suffering and the realization of supreme joy.

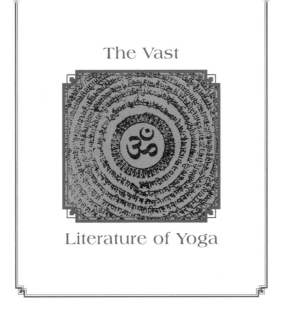

# The Vast

## Literature of Yoga

The teaching of yoga has always relied upon an oral tradition, directly passed on from guru to disciple.[13] Yet, apart from its oral orientation, the yoga tradition has extensive literature, extending into thousands of books primarily written in Sanskrit. This yoga literature is perhaps the largest and oldest spiritual literature in the world.

## Yoga Darshana and the Yoga Sutras ☸

Besides the general meaning of yoga as inner practices to achieve union with the divine, there is a more specific meaning of yoga as one of the systems of Indian philosophy. This *Yoga Darshana*, as it is known in Sanskrit, is one of the six schools of Vedic philosophy that build their authority on the Vedas, Upanishads, and Bhagavad Gita.[14]

Many scholars inaccurately call these six Vedic schools "the six schools of Indian philosophy." Classical Indian philosophy had eleven main schools: six Vedic, four Buddhist, and one Jain. Numerous later schools of Indian philosophy also exist.

We have already mentioned the most commonly known text on yoga, the Yoga Sutras of Patanjali, most likely dating from around 300 BCE. Many commentaries on this text exist, the most important being the ancient edition of Vyasa, which explains the Yoga Sutras in great detail.

While yoga as one of the six systems and as a general term are related, it is important to discriminate between the two. All Vedic systems and many non-Vedic systems in India use yogic methods of asana, pranayama, mantra, and meditation, which were never regarded as belonging to any particular system. But not all emphasize the Yoga Sutras or agree with all of its statements or philosophical orientation. Even many yoga traditions, such as Hatha Yoga, depart from Patanjali's philosophy on some points.[15] The Yoga Darshana also has

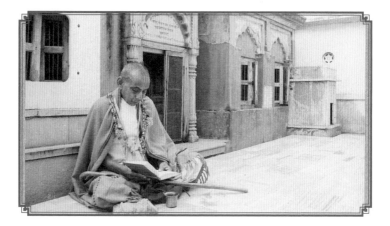

several formulations other than that of Patanjali and existed long before him.

The traditional founder of Yoga Darshana is usually said to be a figure named Hiranyagarbha, who is connected to Vedic mantras and sometimes identified with Lord Brahma or the cosmic creator. The Mahabharata, which contains the Bhagavad Gita, states, "Hiranyagarbha is the knower of yoga; there is not one more ancient."[16] Hiranyagabha, which means "the golden embryo," is a name for the sun god in Vedic texts, referring to the divine light of consciousness.[17] Many yogic teachings are said to derive from the sun god under different names. Vasishta, the greatest of the Vedic seers, to whom a number of yogic texts are ascribed, is mentioned as the main successor to Hiranyagarbha.[18]

Patanjali was a great compiler, not the founder, of the yoga system. So we should not reduce yoga to Patanjali or the Yoga Sutras, however important his compilation may be. Moreover, Patanjali is honored as an incarnation of Lord Sesha, the serpent on which Lord Vishnu rests. Patanjali himself refers to *Ishvara*, or God, as the original teacher of yoga.[19] In fact, the divine is the real teacher behind all the other teachers and incarnations of this spiritual art.

## The Bhagavad Gita, the Supreme Teaching of Yoga ✿

The most famous of the Yoga Shastras, or authoritative texts on yoga, is the Bhagavad Gita, spoken by Sri Krishna. Krishna is called *Yogeshvara*, or the "Lord of Yoga," and said to be the avatar, or divine originator, of yoga. In the Bhagavad Gita, Krishna states that he taught the ancient yoga to the sun god, Vivasvan, who then taught it to Manu, the legendary first king and law giver, who then taught it

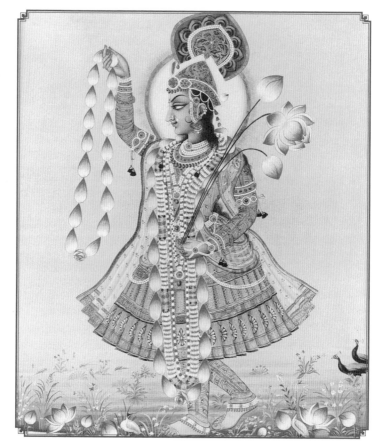

to mankind.[20] Krishna is said to have taken many births to
sustain the yoga teaching in the world.[21]

Each chapter of the Bhagavad Gita is related to a particular
yoga or means of union with the divine. The Gita teaches
the yogas of devotion and knowledge but also mentions the
importance of pranayama, pratyahara, mantra, meditation,
and samadhi, using similar terms to those found later in the

Yoga Sutras. Overall, the Gita takes an integral approach, combining all the main approaches to yoga and harmonizing them. While the Yoga Sutras is a collection of short axioms that does not explain anything in detail, the Gita thoroughly covers all aspects of yoga. Therefore the best way to study the Yoga Sutras is along with the Bhagavad Gita.

The Bhagavad Gita occurs in the context of a much longer text called the Mahabharata, which contains many other important yoga teachings. Most notable are the Moksha Dharma Parva, taught by the great guru Bhishma, and the Anu Gita. These sections tell stories of ancient yogis and their powers. They also call their teachings Yoga Shastras, or authoritative yoga texts.[22] Like other ancient texts, they speak of Hiranyagarbha as the founder of the yoga system.

Besides the Mahabharata is a related set of literature called the Puranas, a vast volume of books related to various deities, such as Shiva, Vishnu, the goddess, and Ganesha. Yoga is one of their common topics and is covered in detail, as in the Mahabharata and Bhagavad Gita. Some Puranas contain special sections on particular yoga topics such as mantra, pranayama, and meditation.

## Yoga and the Upanishads ✵

The Bhagavad Gita is said to represent the essence of an earlier set of teachings called the Upanishads. Because the prime focus of the Gita is yoga practice, one can conclude that the essence of the Upanishads is also yoga. The Upanishadic teaching, called Vedanta, meaning "the end or summit of the Vedas," like yoga, emphasizes the unity of the individual self and the universal self. In fact, Vedanta explains this teaching of unity in great detail, much more than in the Yoga Sutras, which are more practically oriented.

The Upanishads contain many teachings relative to yoga, particularly on meditation, devotion, mantra, and self-inquiry.[23] The Katha Upanishad is particularly considered an authoritative yoga text.[24] The Shvetashvatara Upanishad also covers yoga, using Vedic teachings and mantras for this purpose.[25] Additionally, there is a later set of Yoga Upanishads that contains much information about yogic practices of all types.

Yajnavalkya, the most famous of the Upanishadic sages, is renowned as a great yogi. The Brihadaranyaka, perhaps the oldest and longest of the classical Upanishads, is attributed to him. Later yogic texts such as the Brihad Yogi Yajnavalkya go back to him.

## Vedic Yoga ❋

The Upanishads are considered the essential or secret teaching of the Vedas. As such, one would have to regard yoga as vital to the Vedic approach. The Vedas, of which the mantra section of the Rig Veda is the longest and most important, are considered the ultimate basis of yoga, a term mentioned in several places therein. Manu, the famous original man or flood figure of Hindu thought and prime teacher of the Vedas, is also said to have been a great yogi. He is thought to have used his yoga power to reestablish human culture at the end of the great flood.[26]

Vasishta is usually regarded as the foremost of the *rishis*, or Vedic seers, to whom most of the seventh book of the Rig Veda is ascribed. He is believed to have received the ancient yoga from Hiranyagarbha. Later yoga texts, such as the famous Yoga Vasishta and Vasishta Samhita, are ascribed to the Vasishta line. Vasishta is portrayed as the teacher of Lord Rama, the avatar before Krishna, who learned all the secrets of yoga from him.

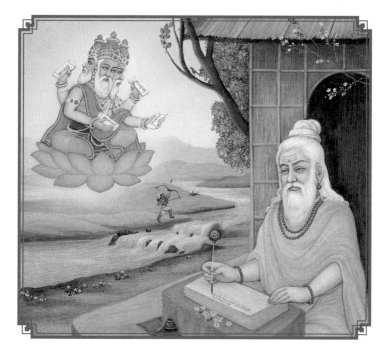

The Vedas specifically are texts of Mantra Yoga, dealing with divine sound as a means of self-realization. Important Vedic mantras such as Gayatri mantra of the rishi Vishvamitra,[27] the Mrityunjaya mantra of the rishi Vasishta,[28] and the Hamsa mantra of the rishi Vamadeva[29] have been commonly used and extolled in yogic teachings throughout the centuries and are still commonly used today.

The Mantra Yoga of the Vedas connects to Bhakti Yoga, the yoga of devotion. The Vedas consist primarily of hymns of praise to the divine in the form of different deities, including calling upon the divine as father, mother, brother, sister, friend, and master. They stress the importance of *namas*, or devotional surrender, and the use of divine names.

On an outer level, the Vedas are texts of Karma Yoga, prescribing special rituals for both physical and spiritual welfare. The Vedic ritual is a sophisticated practice, using special offerings into a sacred fire to invoke higher spiritual influences directly into this material plane. Vedic rituals are famous in India for their power to promote peace, sanctify human actions, and remove negative influences from society. They are still widely performed today, and some groups in the West now also offer them.

Vedic rituals are called *yajnas*, or sacrifices. Yoga is believed to have arisen as the inner aspect of the Vedic sacrifice, in which one offers speech, mind, and prana into the divine flame of awareness dwelling in the heart, which is identified with Vishnu.[30] In this regard, all aspects of the Vedic sacrifice have inner counterparts. Similarly yoga is best performed as a sacred ritual, an offering of ourselves to the higher reality.

## Yoga and the Sects of Hindu Dharma

Traditionally the Hindu belief systems are divided into five sects: the Shaivite, Vaishnava, Shakti, Ganapata, and Saura, according to whether they primarily worship Shiva, Vishnu, the goddess, Ganesha, or the sun god (Surya). All these sects emphasize various yoga practices, which are explained mainly in the Puranas that relate to these deities but occur in other texts as well, including special Upanishads relative to them.

Like Krishna, Shiva is honored as the *Yogeshvara*, or the great "Lord of Yoga." He is the main deity of the great Himalayan yogis, and he originated many yoga traditions. The goddess, or Shakti as Uma, is honored as the greatest of the yoginis and as the very power of yoga. Shiva and Shakti are the deities of many Inner Yoga practices of pranayama, mantra, and Tantra. The goddess is regarded as the power of yoga. Many great modern yogis of India, such as Ramakrishna and Sri Aurobindo, were specifically worshippers of the goddess.

Vishnu as Krishna is also the great avatar of yoga, as we have mentioned. Vishnu's consort, Lakshmi, is called Yogamaya, or "the power of yoga." Other forms of Vishnu, such as Rama, are closely connected to different yoga teachings,[31] as is the Narayana form of Vishnu. Hanuman, the monkey companion of Rama, is often portrayed as a great yogi.

The son of Shiva and the goddess, Ganesha, who has the head of an elephant, is also lauded as a great teacher of yoga. He is worshipped to remove any obstacles from yoga practice and to provide the wisdom to proceed. He is specifically a deity of the root chakra and gives great mantric powers as well.

Surya, the sun god, representing the divine light, is considered the founder of many Vedic and yogic traditions. The Vedic mantras are said to dwell in the rays of the sun. Special yoga pranayamas follow the courses of the sun, moon, planets and signs of the zodiac.[32]

## Tantric Yoga

Tantra is regarded as the third layer of Hindu teachings, after the Vedas and Puranas. Tantra closely follows the deities and practices of the Puranas. Tantric Yoga is mainly the worship of Shiva and Shakti as the deities of yoga.

In the West, the sexual side of Tantric Yoga has been emphasized, but sacred sex is just one aspect of Tantric teaching, which covers all the paths of yoga. More specifically, Tantric Yoga emphasizes the use of deities, mantras, and yantras as part of its path to self-realization. Tantric Yoga also employs special rituals and use of sacred sites in nature.

Many medieval and modern yoga sects from India are Tantric, including the traditions of Hatha Yoga and Siddha Yoga. They are highly honored in Tibetan circles as well. They mainly follow Adi Nath, Lord Shiva, who is also considered the original teacher of Hatha Yoga.[33]

## Buddhism and Yoga ✻

Buddhism has yogic teachings, particularly in the Tantric traditions followed in Tibet. It expounds pranayama, mantra, and the worship of deities, much like Hindu Tantra. Like classical yoga, Buddhist Yoga emphasizes the yoga of meditation.

The main differences between Hindu and Buddhist yogas are philosophical. Buddhism is a nontheistic tradition and does not recognize a creator behind the universe, something to which Vedantic philosophy affords great importance. According to Buddhism, karma creates the world, and no god is necessary.

Buddhism also does not accept the ultimacy of a higher self (Atma or Purusha) but teaches the importance of the nonself (Anatma), while yoga and Vedanta emphasize the Atman or Purusha. Similarly, Buddhism does not posit any absolute or Brahman behind the manifest world, such as the Upanishads laud. Buddhism emphasizes the voidness of all things and the reality of mind only.

However, although traditional Buddhism rejects yoga, Samkhya, and Vedantic teachings on certain philosophical points, it shares with them many common ideas and practices, such as the theory of karma and the practice of using mantras such as OM.

## Jain Yoga ✣

The Jain tradition of India also has its great yogis, ascetics, saints, poets, and scientists. Jain Yoga is highly ascetic and emphasizes self-control. Its main principle is ahimsa or nonviolence. Yet it also uses mantra, meditation, and the whole range of yoga practices.

## Modern Yoga and Its Literature ✣

The modern literature on yoga is now very extensive and can be found in most of the main languages of the world. Some of this literature consists of translations of traditional yoga texts such as the Yoga Sutras. Another portion comes from modern yoga teachers of India, many of whom, like Sri Aurobindo or Swami Shivananda, were prolific writers in the English language.

Recently a large amount of literature on yoga asanas has developed, both by Indian and Western yoga teachers. It includes books, videos, and classes aimed mainly at yoga asanas, which dominate the popular yoga scene. Meanwhile, only a few books about the deeper, or inner, yoga have come out in recent years. This means that the yoga student has a lot of information to choose from, though not always a clear orientation to the higher teachings.

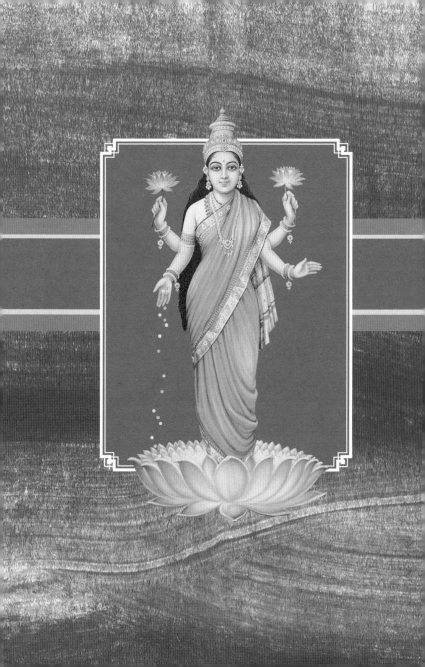

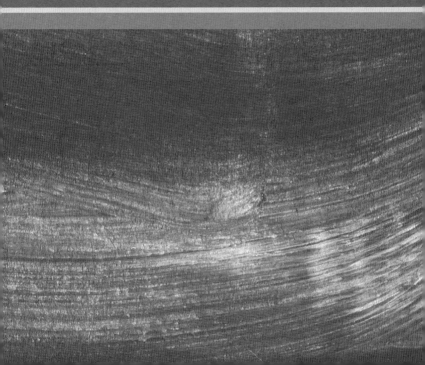

PART TWO

# THE GREATER
# PRACTICES OF YOGA

# The Integral System

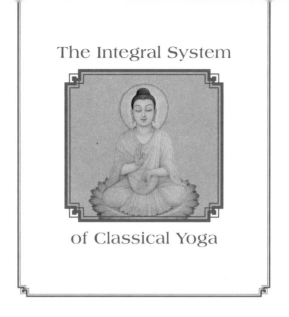

## of Classical Yoga

We have defined yoga as a comprehensive spiritual path including asana, pranayama, mantra, and meditation, but how do we bring these diverse aspects of yoga into play in our own practice?

The Yoga Sutras outlines a yoga of eight limbs, or Ashtanga Yoga.[34] While there are many other formulations in the Yoga Sutras and other texts, this remains probably the best and most comprehensive model for yoga practice as a whole. It is also called Raja Yoga, or "the royal path," because it provides a way to relate yoga to all aspects of life. Many other yogic texts stress these same principal factors of yoga practice. They are not unique to Patanjali, though his formulation of them is the best known.[35]

# The Eight Limbs of Yoga ☀

1. **Yama**: *yogic attitudes and observances*

2. **Niyama**: *yogic lifestyle practices*

3. **Asana**: *yoga postures*

4. **Pranayama**: *yogic breathing and energy work*

5. **Pratyahara**: *internalization of the mind and senses*

6. **Dharana**: *concentration*

7. **Dhyana**: *meditation*

8. **Samadhi**: *absorption or unity consciousness*

The yamas and niyamas provide a yogic attitude, system of values, and lifestyle that sustain the practice of yoga at a spiritual level. Asana is the yoga of the physical body, affording harmony and balance to the body, its systems, tissues, and organs. Pranayama is the yoga of the breath and vital energy, improving and harmonizing our life force. Pratyahara is the yoga of the senses, showing how to use our senses in the optimal manner to open up to higher influences and reduce disturbing ones.

Dharana is the yoga of the outer mind, designed to cultivate attention and focus to our awareness. Dhyana is the yoga of the inner mind, teaching us how to hold the mind steady in a receptive state of meditation. Samadhi is the yoga of the inner heart, through which our higher bliss and peace can arise.

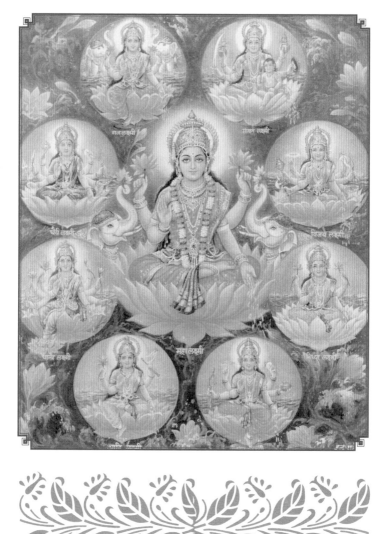

## Outer Yoga and Inner Yoga ✺

These eight limbs of yoga are more simply divided into the "outer limbs of yoga" (*bahir anga*) and the "inner limbs of yoga" (*antar anga*). We can call these two the Outer Yoga and the Inner Yoga.

The Outer Yoga consists of the first five limbs, which extend to the realm of the senses. The Inner Yoga consists of the last three limbs: dharana, dhyana, and samadhi, which relate to the mind, awareness, and meditation in the broader sense.

The Outer Yoga is designed to prepare us for the Inner Yoga. For inner awareness to develop, it is necessary to first bring harmony and balance to the outer mind, body, and senses. The Outer Yoga aims at our physical and psychological well-being. The Inner Yoga aims at self-realization beyond body and mind. The Outer Yoga is often called Hatha Yoga, though its higher component directs us to the Inner Yoga as well. The Inner Yoga is often called Raja Yoga, though its foundation includes the Outer Yoga.

Most popular forms of yoga today belong to the Outer Yoga. They involve mainly physical movements, an extensive asana workout, with perhaps some breath work, a little chanting, and a few minutes of meditation. Whereas the Outer Yoga is the current face of modern yoga, we should remember that the Inner Yoga is the real purpose of traditional yoga.

# Yoga Practice, Discrimination, and Nonattachment ☙

The main factors behind yoga practice are defined in its vast literature. The primary term for yoga practice is *Abhyasa*, which means "dwelling over" something. Abhyasa relates to two factors of *Viveka*, or discriminating insight, and *Vairagya*, or nonattachment.[36]

**Viveka** refers to the ability of the higher mind to discern the true from the false, the real from the unreal, the inner from the outer, and the eternal from the transient. While this may sound like an easy thing to do, it is actually very difficult because our minds, senses, and prana naturally draw us into the external world.

**Vairagya** is the ability to refrain from involving ourselves in external affairs, to avoid identifications, compulsions, opinions, likes, and dislikes. This also is not easy because we have so many personal and social concerns in our ordinary lives. But we can achieve it by degrees, through consistently directing our awareness within.

On this foundation, we will study the eight limbs of yoga, one by one, examining in detail the role of each and its application.

# YAMAS & NIYAMAS:

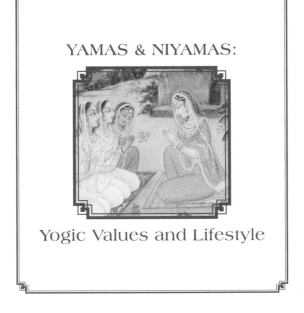

## Yogic Values and Lifestyle

Yoga is a conscious way of living that rests upon a particular set of values, attitudes, and observances. A yogic lifestyle can probably best be described as a dharmic way of life, following the natural and spiritual laws behind the universe for the benefit of all beings. These principles, the dharmas of yoga practice, are not mere commandments to be followed mechanically. They are based upon the idea that all life should be respected, and they must be adapted individually, according to time, place, and circumstance.

For example, take the principle of *ahimsa*, or nonharming, which is the first principle of yoga. No creature in the universe wants to be harmed. We ourselves do not want to be harmed. Therefore, if we want to live in harmony, avoiding harming others is the first thing to consider, no matter what religion or philosophy we espouse in our outer lives.

Yoga begins with its lifestyle principles or dharmic values. These constitute the yamas and niyamas as the first two of the eight limbs of yoga.

## The Five Yamas ✵

The five yamas are primary yogic values, principles, and observances. They mainly consist of forms of self-regulation. A yogic lifestyle is a disciplined life, controlled not by violence or force but by a higher aspiration.

*1. Ahimsa* is often translated as nonviolence, but it is not just about avoiding violence. It is ensuring that our lifestyle causes minimal damage to the world around us, and it actually aims to reduce the amount of harm that occurs.

Yoga wishes happiness for all beings and respects the sacred nature of all life. This is reflected in the yogic prayers and chants for universal peace. Ahimsa usually includes a vegetarian diet because meat eating is one of the most obvious ways that we unnecessarily hurt other creatures.

*2. Satya* is truthfulness in the deepest sense of the word. We should be true to ourselves and others, and speak the truth. Otherwise, we cannot pursue the Inner Yoga, which is a pursuit of truth. Satya does not mean merely avoiding lies but promoting the cause of truth in the world in our actions and expressions.

*3. Asteya* is nonstealing, not only at a physical level but also at a psychological level. We should not take what does not belong to us. We should not take credit for what we have not actually done. In the highest sense, nothing belongs to us. We are only stewards of nature's resources.

4. *Brahmacharya* is a particularly difficult term for us to understand today. It is often translated as celibacy, though for married people it means faithfulness in marriage. Brahmacharya refers to the proper usage of our sexual energy, which has a great power not only for creation but also for destruction if applied carelessly. Unless we use this energy in a conscious manner, much pain and suffering will be caused in the world.

5. *Aparigraha* is a hard term to translate, but perhaps nonpossessiveness is the best equivalent. Not accumulating any unnecessary possessions outwardly or inwardly is aparigraha. The mental side is important. Even if we may not physically possess something, we may still hold or cling to it in our thoughts and emotions.

## The Niyamas ✼

> The niyamas are the five basic attitudes behind yoga practice. They are ways of holding, conserving, and internalizing our energies.

1. *Tapas* refers to the inner heat or fire of yoga that can develop the higher capacities within us. It is not an enforced or military discipline but, like the inspiration of an artist, arises from our own inner seeking. It includes the austerity or self-control necessary to turn our awareness within.

2. *Svadhyaya* means the study of what relates to oneself. It is sometimes called self-study. In the broader sense, it means to fulfill one's *svadharma*, or individual dharma. This includes understanding one's unique psychophysical nature and the particular orientation to the divine inherent within oneself, giving it a devotional component.[37]

*3. Ishvara pranidhana* appears throughout the Yoga Sutras as a prime principle of devotion to the divine presence. It is not simply a theological belief. It is a consecration of our energy to the cosmic power.

*4. Saucha* refers to purity in the broadest sense of the term, purity of body, speech, and mind. This means cleanliness of the body and mind. A vegetarian diet is often considered one of the main factors of physical purity.

*5. Santosha* is inner contentment, a principle often forgotten when we view yoga as some form of effort-based austerity. Yoga arises from a pursuit of inner peace and happiness, not a seeking of external rewards, titles, or fame. We should be content with what we have outwardly, finding our true happiness within.

The first three niyamas—tapas, svadhyaya, and Ishvara pranidhana—also stand alone as Kriya Yoga, the practice of yoga in the more general sense.[38] All eight limbs of yoga can be employed as part of these three. They serve to increase the heat of yoga, to promote self-awareness, and to help us dedicate ourselves to the higher cosmic powers.

# Yamas and Niyamas and Karma Yoga ⚛

The yamas and niyamas form the basis of Karma Yoga, the yoga of selfless action. They show us how to behave in the world in a conscious manner that is itself a yoga practice. All yoga begins with Karma Yoga, which is action done as a service to others and as a form of worship of the divine.

Being a karma yogi means that we regard all action as sacred. We act with consciousness and respect for the greater universe around us and for the welfare of all creatures. This does not mean that we must necessarily become socially or politically active but that we should always act for the greater good. In this way, Karma Yoga takes us beyond karma. It makes our action into a force of liberation, not only for ourselves but also for others.

Karma Yoga is not just what we do but reflects our attitude. It requires that our outer actions be performed from a peaceful state of mind that wishes all creatures well, even our enemies. Karma Yoga is *sattvic* action, action taken to reduce harm and create understanding. Such yogic action can confront difficulty, or even evil, but does so from a center of inner peace that is the real power of transformation, whereas ordinary social and political action usually causes additional polarization between groups of people, thus resulting in further violence and hatred.

To be a yogic activist is to promote integration in society by bringing us back into harmony with nature and the true divine presence that transcends all outer forms and institutions. To reach this level of yogic action is a very high achievement for the soul. It occurs when we give up the "ego of action" and let the higher powers work through us.

# ASANA:

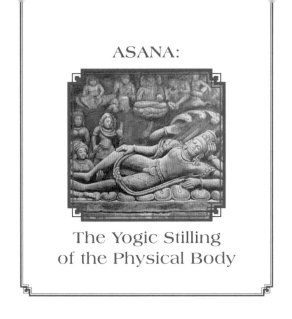

## The Yogic Stilling
## of the Physical Body

In traditional yoga, asana is used primarily to prepare the body for deeper yoga practices. It is not an end in itself but forms the foundation for the rest of yoga. The term asana means literally a "seat" in Sanskrit, so asana indicates preparing the seat for yoga practice. Traditional yoga aims at developing sitting postures so that we can practice pranayama and meditation without physical distractions or discomfort. Other yoga postures and movements are designed to help relax the body so that a sitting posture is easy to maintain.

Asana is designed to develop *sattva guna*, the quality of calmness in the body, and to counter *rajo-guna*, the quality of agitation. This means that real asana practice includes a fair amount of stillness and inaction, not of an enforced nature, but one that arises from releasing stress and letting go of the ego. Asana helps put the body into a state of nondoing so that our inner consciousness can come forth. This means that asana is more about the reduction of physical movement than the development of movement.

The best sitting postures are *padmasana* (lotus pose), *siddhasana* (perfection pose) and *vajrasana* (diamond pose). However, any comfortable pose (*sukhasana*) can be used, even if it requires sitting in a chair. The goal of asana practice is to be able to sit calmly, not to twist the body into difficult poses.

## Asana and Exercise

Yoga asana is an ideal form of exercise because it can relieve stress, remove toxins, and reduce tension, as well as make us physically stronger and more flexible. Many other forms of exercise, despite providing a good workout, increase tension in the muscles, bones, and joints, thus causing more stress in the nervous system and mind.

Asana teaches us to slow down our bodily movements to help calm the mind, senses, and nervous system. It helps us reduce excessive activity, so the body does not lose energy and can rejuvenate itself from within. It changes the way our physical energy works and moves, allowing it to become steady, concentrated, and at peace.

Yoga asanas are not only good for the young but also for the elderly. Many of the problems of aging, such as arthritis, originate in the bones and can be reduced by regular asana practice. For the young, yoga postures have a calming effect and reduce hyperactivity, agitation, and distraction.

## Asana and Prana ✸

Many great yogis learned their asanas by following the inner *prana*, or vital energy, that came to them during meditation. Asana is not just about achieving the ideal form of one posture or another. It is about allowing the prana, or cosmic life energy, to flow through and revitalize us. Prana has a higher intelligence that aligns the body with the currents of universal life and consciousness.

Yoga asanas should flow like the breath rather than serve as a series of specifically defined movements. We should remember to move with and through prana in our asana practice, letting the energy unfold. Even sitting poses should be held with the "fullness of prana" rather than by personal effort alone.

## Asana and Awareness ✸

Like all aspects of yoga, asana requires a conscious approach. It is essential in asana practice to remain aware and alert, not simply of our body and its structure but of the entire movement of our thought and breath. This requires putting the mind into a calm, witnessing state and making the body into a vehicle for meditation.

Real asana is done with a higher awareness of one's inner being. We should remain aware of our higher nature and our connection with the divine during asana practice rather than worry about how our bodies look.

# An Asana Yogi ✤

Today's image of a yogi is largely that of an asana yogi, one who is adept at a great variety of yoga asanas and possesses extraordinary physical flexibility. But a real asana yogi can sit quietly, relaxed and aware, connected to the cosmic mind and prana without feeling a need to move or even talk. He or she does not necessarily have to be good at difficult yoga postures; otherwise a gymnast would automatically be a yogi. True asana practice means to be seated in one's own nature, abiding in the inner heart. Then, not only the body but our entire being will become part of the asana and its stillness.

Try to develop a comfortable sitting pose and use it to dive into deep meditation. A real asana expert can hold a steady sitting pose comfortably for at least one hour. This is the main perfection of asana sought in classical yoga. Remember that yoga practice does not end with asana but only begins with it. If you stop your practice with asana, you may have a good workout, but you have not yet done real yoga, which rests upon integrating body, mind, and spirit.

It is good to practice yoga asanas for half an hour or more in the morning and a similar period later in the day. But one need not overdo asana practice. It should be done gently, with detachment. The purpose of asana is to help us let go of body consciousness, not increase it.

Classical yoga teaches us that too much fixation on asana can even become an obstacle to higher yoga practice. This occurs when our asana practice results in the creation of more body consciousness rather than less. Remember that the body has a certain dullness or heaviness to it. If we dwell too much on the physical, the mind tends to get pulled down. Practice asana with lightness, as if your body were made of light and energy.

# PRANAYAMA:

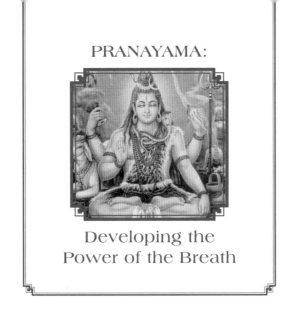

## Developing the
## Power of the Breath

We all seek more energy in life. But we usually look outside ourselves, seeking emotional needs from other people. Alternatively, yoga teaches us how to develop more energy inside ourselves, one that doesn't require depending upon anyone external to receive it. This frees us from outer energy needs and provides us with unlimited internal resources to draw upon for our true happiness.

*Prana* is the yogic term for our connection through the breath with the unlimited and inexhaustible universal life force. Prana is the vital energy that enables both the body and mind to function. Yogic breathing exercises are an important means of developing prana. They are the main factor of pranayama, the fourth of the eight limbs of yoga.

Prana is the power or the shakti of yoga. It is through prana, or the internal life force, that the internal process of yoga unfolds. Yoga is not a matter of mere personal effort but of moving with the cosmic forces. The breath is an indication not only of the fact that we are alive but also of our connection to a greater formless reality, indicated by the air element and extending into infinite space. Note that whenever we make an important effort in life, we usually take a deep breath first.

For higher yoga practices, one needs more energy, or prana, for the mind and consciousness, which is facilitated by yogic deep breathing, or pranayama. Yet we can also use this increased prana for physical healing or to help us do whatever we really want to accomplish in life.

Prana is an important subject of many yoga teachings, including how the prana relates to the channels, nadis, and chakras of both the physical and the subtle energy bodies.[39] Traditional yoga practice centers on prana, affording it much more emphasis than asana, which is viewed as a vehicle for releasing prana.

The breath is unique among our bodily functions because we can breathe either automatically or voluntarily. We can exercise our breath, just as we can exercise our body. In this process we can work our entire respiratory tract and energy field as a whole.

## Important Pranayama Techniques ❧

There are a number of important, powerful pranayama techniques in classical yoga. These are usually done in sitting postures, but some can be performed in other postures as well. In all yogic forms of pranayama, one should ground the breath in the belly or even in the base of the spine. This allows one to breathe with the entire body.

Yogic breathing usually emphasizes drawing in the breath while making an audible sound at the back of the throat, which is called *ujjayi pranayama* in Sanskrit.

Other yoga techniques consist of rapid deep breathing, with forceful exhalation or inhalation through the nostrils, the most common of which are *bhastrika* and *kapalabhati*, which open the sinuses in the head and stimulate the brain and senses.

Certain pranayamas, particularly breathing with the mouth, are cooling and calming in nature, notably *shitali*, when one breathes out through the mouth with the tongue curled.

The most common and useful yogic form of pranayama is alternate nostril breathing (called *nadi shodana* in Sanskrit), which is a means of purifying the channels of the subtle body and the nervous system. Long ago, yogis understood the balance of right and left, male and female, and fiery and watery energies in the body. They learned to use the breath to balance these, closing one nostril at a time for inhalation and exhalation. Once prana is balanced, it can take a quantum leap to a higher level of manifestation, opening up new vistas of energy for us.

It is best to have a yoga teacher instruct you in these forms of pranayama because they are subtle and need to be done correctly. Yet all of us can benefit from practicing pranayama for at least half an hour a day, particularly in the morning, to open up our energy and stimulate the mind and senses.

## Prana, Sound, and Mantra ❧

Speech, which uses the outgoing breath, is said in yogic texts to be manifest prana. Prana, which we take in through inhalation, is considered unmanifest or primal sound. Because of this connection, pranayama and mantra are often used together to link prana and speech, and then prana and mind through speech.

Inhale gently and deeply, mentally repeating the mantric sound OM, and feel your energy rise from the base of your spine to the top of your head, expanding along the way. Exhale, mentally repeating the mantra sound HUM (pronounced "hoom"), and feel your energy come forth with the ability to express itself in speech or action. This practice will give you a sense of how mantra and breath go together.

The breath has a natural hissing sound, as we find in *s* and *h* sounds. Another pranayama method is to listen to the natural sound of the breath SO upon inhalation, and HAM (with "A" as the vowel sound "uh" in *the*) upon exhalation, letting your breath naturally deepen in the process. In this way, mind, speech, and prana get automatically attuned to higher frequencies. You can also practice this natural sound of the breath in pranayama.

## Pranayama and Meditation ❦

Steadiness in meditation requires a concentrated mental focus, which is supported by a concentrated power of the prana. Through pranayama, we concentrate our energy and draw it inward, creating an additional power to stabilize the mind. So, pranayama itself is a kind of prana meditation.

We not only think with our minds but also with our prana, which means with our life force, will, intention, emotion, and instinct. The more we bring prana into our meditation, the more depth it has, and the capacity for internal transformation is greater.

## Prana Yoga ✦

Through the practice of pranayama, you can become a prana yogi, one who is united with prana as the cosmic life force.

Breath and mind are connected like the two wings of a bird. The breath reflects our thoughts and emotions. When the mind is disturbed, the breath is disturbed, and when the breath is disturbed, the mind is disturbed. For example, fear makes us forget to breathe, and anger makes us breathe harder.

When we calm and release the breath, our mental and emotional stress gets relieved in this process. Through Prana Yoga you can learn to breathe your problems away. Whenever a disturbing emotion arises in your mind, gather its energy upon inhalation, and release the negative emotion on exhalation.

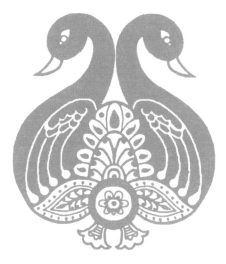

# PRATYAHARA:

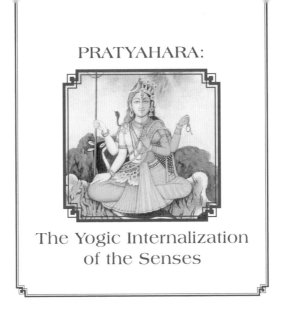

## The Yogic Internalization of the Senses

Pratyahara is known as "the forgotten limb" of yoga. Few yoga teachers today know what it is or include it in their classes, though it has been regarded as the most important aspect of classical yoga.

Pratyahara is often regarded as a kind of control or suppression of the senses. Because we live in a highly sensate culture, with its mass media, computers, pop music, and so on, pratyahara might seem out of place. However, pratyahara is really about the right use of the senses, just as asana concerns the right use of the body and pranayama the right use of the breath. Pratyahara is crucial not only to yoga but also to right living in general, particularly in this media age of sensory stimulation.

Pratyahara serves as the bridge between the Outer Yoga of physical postures and the Inner Yoga of meditation. To move from the Outer Yoga's focus on the external world to the Inner Yoga's focus on consciousness, we must first turn our energy within. Pratyahara concerns this internalization of energy that is necessary not only for meditation but also for any deep healing. If we can internalize our energy, we can also strengthen our immune systems and de-stress our nerves, as well as open up higher levels of awareness.

The way we use our senses is the basis for how we conduct our lives. The senses are our gateways to the outer world and its various influences. Most importantly, the senses provide a subtle form of nutrition for the mind. In the yoga system, our five types of sensory impressions are regarded as the five subtle elements and correspond to the gross elements:

| Senses | Elements |
|--------|----------|
| Sight | Fire |
| Sound | Ether |
| Smell | Earth |
| Touch | Air |
| Taste | Water |

Just as the gross elements build the body through the food we eat, the subtle elements build the mind through the sensory impressions we take in. Just as we should consider the nutritional quality of our food for the health of our bodies, we should consider the nutritional quality of our sensory impressions if we want our mind to be healthy and balanced.

In the modern world we suffer not just from sensory overload but from an even deeper sensory deprivation. Though we are bombarded with sensory stimuli, these are largely of a dulling nature, mainly bright colors and loud noises that desensitize us to the greater range of nature's beauties.

We can compare junk impressions with junk food. Those who live on junk food, even if overweight, actually suffer from malnutrition, not having the adequate vitamins, minerals, and prana in their food to provide steady energy and good tissue formation. Similarly our minds are overweight from a diet of media-based impressions that are much like junk food, heavy but not nourishing. The bright lights and dramatic events of the media blind us. We cannot simply be quiet in the woods or mountains. Nature might be considered a natural pratyahara. Without it, our energies remain distracted and out of balance.

Pratyahara concerns developing the natural power of our senses. This also helps us discover our inner senses, the ability to see lights and hear sounds within our own minds. These inner vibrations are not simply hallucinations but forms of contact with the higher worlds. Pratyahara involves cultivating these inner senses.

Another aspect of pratyahara is giving our senses a rest. Like any organs or muscles, our senses can be overstimulated and overworked. Pratyahara means letting our outer senses relax so that their energy and acuity can be renewed. Most of us suffer from worn-out senses. By turning the senses within, their vitality can be restored.

## Simple Methods of Pratyahara ❧

There are many simple methods of pratyahara that are essential to a peaceful, healthy, and happy life.

### Keeping Silent, or Mauna

Not speaking is one of the best forms of pratyahara. Speech is our most active motor organ and the main site through which we lose energy in life. Our constant chatter makes our prana disperse so that our minds become dull. Keeping silent allows our energy to turn within and give us strength. Silence of speech also aids in calming and silencing the mind. Many great yogis have practiced not speaking for extended periods. Some have even given up speaking altogether. Try not speaking for one day a week and see how it deepens your energy and awareness.

## Pranayama

Pranayama itself can be a very effective form of pratyahara. To practice this, take the energy gained from deep breathing and hold it inside. This way, we follow the prana within, taking the mind and senses inward along with the breath. The energy of prana can be retained in the heart chakra or in any of the chakras for this purpose.

## Asana

Asana is natural pratyahara of the motor organs, in which our arms and legs slow down and cease their movement. This asana pratyahara occurs in any posture wherein we achieve stillness, particularly sitting poses maintained silently for long periods. A calm body allows the mind to be calm as well.

## Closing the Senses

Perhaps the most classical method of pratyahara is to close the eyes. With a technique called *Yoni Mudra*, one can cut off the other senses as well, using the fingers to close the eyes, ears, nostrils, and mouth. When our outer senses are no longer active, our higher inner faculties can come forth.

## Engaging the Inner Senses

Engaging the inner senses consists of closing the eardrums and listening to the inner sounds, and closing the eyes and gazing into the inner light. Yogis see inner lights called *jyoti* and hear inner sounds called *nada*. Strong pranayama practice can cause these currents to come forth, as does any steady concentration of the mind. Learn to open your inner senses, so you can experience the worlds within your own mind.

## Hiking

Even a simple natural activity such as hiking can be an active form of pratyahara. This requires remaining silent while hiking, and extending our awareness through our senses into nature, noting the nuances of color, sound, shape, texture, and movement that we might otherwise miss. In fact, a kind of pratyahara happens whenever we immerse our minds in nature, even when gardening.

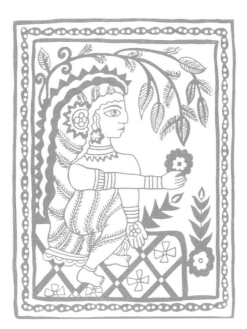

# The Inner Yoga

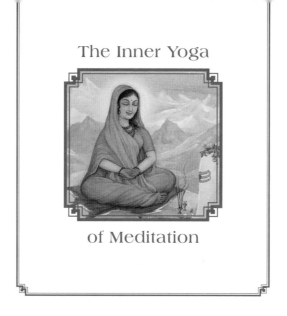

## of Meditation

Meditation is probably the greatest adventure in life, unfolding vast new vistas of knowledge, awareness, and joy. It affords us the maximum self-discovery and greatest scope for exploring the real nature of the universe. Through deep meditation we can access inner worlds of consciousness that are more glorious and magical than even the subtlest realms of matter and energy being examined by science today.

When we close our eyes, why don't we see these inner realms of beauty and delight? We have not yet learned how to open the inner mind, eyes, and ears to be aware of them. This is what the yoga of meditation allows us to do.

The Inner Yoga, which is the main focus of classical yoga, is primarily the yoga of meditation. It consists of the three higher limbs of yoga: *dharana* (concentration), *dhyana* (reflective meditation) and *samadhi* (unified awareness). In this chapter we will discuss all three because they are closely related and work together. However, yoga does not teach meditation immediately. It first aims to create the right foundation for meditation in our personal lives. Without right preparation, meditation is unlikely to succeed or go very deep.

## The Outer Limbs of Yoga and Meditation ⚜

The yogic lifestyle practices of the yamas and niyamas are the dharmic principles of behavior that sustain a life of meditation. Meditation is not separate from how we live but is the fruit of a life in harmony with nature. First, we must make our daily activities into a field in which meditation can flower. That is what nonharming, truthfulness, and other yogic principles create for us.

Yoga asana is designed to allow us to sit comfortably for long periods of meditation without physical strain. The goal of asana is to make the body a suitable vehicle for meditation. Properly performed, asana is a meditation in motion or a meditation brought into the body itself.

Pranayama creates more energy to be directed within to provide greater power for meditation. Unless we use the extra prana provided by pranayama for meditation, we are not really practicing yoga but are merely giving more energy to the outer mind and ego. Yet without the energy support of pranayama, our meditation may turn into a state of sleep, dullness, or mere blankness.

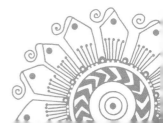

Pratyahara helps us turn our attention and senses within, to internalize the mind for meditation. It uses the senses as instruments for consciousness, awakening their inner and subtle counterparts. All the outer limbs of yoga take us in the direction of meditation. All levels of yoga are a movement in meditation.

## Yogic Meditation ☸

We must always remember that yoga is never just one thing. Yoga is a means of harmonizing all aspects of our lives. *So there is no one yoga meditation technique, any more than there is only one yoga asana or only one yogic form of pranayama.* Yogic forms of meditation have many common elements but also a diversity in their expression.

## Concentration (Dharana) ☸

Yoga describes meditation, in a broader sense, as a threefold process of concentration (*dharana*), reflective meditation (*dhyana*), and unified awareness or absorption (*samadhi*). This means that for meditation to proceed, we must first develop concentration. Without concentration we cannot really meditate, though we may be able to sit quietly and spin in our thoughts.

Many of us get stuck here. We come from a mass-media culture in which our attention jumps from one media stimulus to another every few seconds. We have a difficult time concentrating on anything, particularly the processes of our own minds, which don't provide much entertainment.

The power of attention is a lot like a muscle; if you don't use it, it gets weak and atrophies. Most of us possess an atrophied power of attention. We must develop this power and strengthen it by degrees until we can hold our minds in steady concentration. To achieve this, we must work our attention every day, just as we exercise our bodies regularly.

There are outer tools for developing concentration, such as focusing one's gaze on an external flame from a candle or a ghee lamp. Actually, any natural object can be used for this purpose. There are also inner tools of concentration, such as focusing the mind on the chakras, the breath, or the flame of awareness in the heart.

The key to dharana is being able to consistently direct, fix, and hold one's gaze, whether outwardly or inwardly, on a particular place. Wherever we direct our gaze, our attention automatically follows. The power of dharana resides in the eyes, and dharana helps open the third eye, our inner eye, which can see into infinity.

One important dharana technique is *Shambhavi mudra*, in which we keep our eyes open but direct our gaze within, particularly to the region of the third eye. We can also focus on the third eye with the eyes closed. In this way our concentration becomes steady, and external sensory energies can no longer distract us.

## Meditation (Dhyana) ✹

According to yoga philosophy, the mind has a twofold potential, depending on whether we direct it outwardly or inwardly. If we direct the mind toward the outer world, it gets agitated by desire or distracted by the senses, losing its inherent clarity and peace and compelling us to chase worldly things. However, if we direct the mind within, the mind becomes naturally calm, contemplative, and meditative—happy in its own being and free of external influence. So, in the highest sense meditation is not a technique but the very nature of the internalized mind. Meditation techniques are tools to help us turn and hold the mind within. There are many such techniques using the power of awareness itself or adding mantras, pranayamas, visualizations, and other processes.

In its natural calm state, the mind functions like a mirror to reveal the inner reality of whatever we hold our attention on. The meditative mind can provide us special knowledge of the universe, the subtle worlds, or the deeper dimensions of our own being. Such direct knowledge is very different from that found in books or learned through others. It provides a certainty and sense of eternity in which all our doubts are put to rest.

### Meditating on the Self as the Witness

Probably the most fundamental form of yogic meditation is what is called "taking the attitude of the witness," *sakshi bhava* in Sanskrit. The higher self, or Purusha, is our inner witness, observing but not affected by the fluctuations of the body, mind, and senses. All of us have a sense of this inner witness. It is that part of our nature that remains calm even in the midst of the greatest turmoil, which tells us "this is not as real as it seems to be" or "this too shall pass." If we can cultivate the sense of the witness on a daily basis, we can pursue almost any approach to meditation.

### Yogic Devotional Meditation

Yogic meditation can take a devotional turn as well. In this approach, we meditate upon the divine as present in our hearts, whether as a deity, incarnation (avatar), guru, or anything else that inspires us. We imagine the heart as an eight-petaled lotus in the center of the chest, where the divine dwells at the deepest core of our being.

If we do not want to use a form, we can simply meditate upon the presence of divine love in the heart. We can also meditate upon divine names or mantras of the deities along with their forms. Along with meditation on the deity, we should cultivate surrender to the divine (*Ishvara pranidhana*).

# Yoga and Samadhi, or Unified Awareness

Samadhi is one of the special terms of yoga that refers to a state of absorption in higher awareness, a kind of bliss or inner ecstasy. For many of us, it may seem little more than a yogic high, but it is more like a state of deep and unshakable than any transient euphoria (which usually has its downside as well).

Yoga is frequently defined in terms of samadhi. Yoga as union is samadhi, or absorption in the object with which we seek to unite. Samadhi is a state of meditation so deep that the barriers between yourself and the object of your experience disappear, ultimately including the barrier between yourself and the divine. It is when you feel at one with everything at the core of your being. We have all had such moments of unitary awareness, whether in nature, art, religious experiences, or other ways. Yoga shows us how to cultivate this unitary state so that it becomes the natural condition of our awareness.

### Yogic Samyama

The Yoga Sutras speak of the combined state of dharana, dhyana, and samadhi as *samyama*, which means "total concentration."[40] Samyama is the ability to apply dharana, dhyana, and samadhi at will. It is the total yogic concentration that grants the highest knowledge and power. Most of the third section of the Yoga Sutras discusses the role of samyama and what can be gained by yogic concentration on different objects. This is also the way to the *siddhis*, or "mystic powers" of yoga.

However, the highest samyama is to maintain the state of one's true nature in the heart, which is one with the divine. This takes us beyond the need for any other forms of concentration and grants us the supreme power to be one with all that is.

In the following three sections, we will examine additional approaches to the Inner Yoga of meditation: the yoga of knowledge, the yoga of devotion, and the yoga of energetic practices.

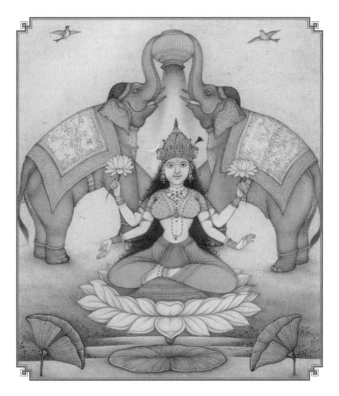

# JNANA YOGA:

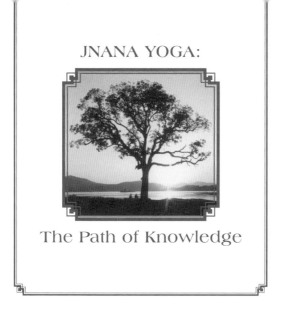

## The Path of Knowledge

The yoga of knowledge is perhaps the most important aspect of the Inner Yoga of meditation. It is often regarded as the highest yoga because it takes us directly to self-realization. The yoga of knowledge exists as part of classical Raja Yoga, or eight-limbed yoga, but also constitutes its own special path of Jnana Yoga.

To develop such inner knowledge requires the appropriate instrument. You cannot know your inner being, which exists beyond time and space, through outer instruments or through a chemical analysis of the body or brain. Such outer tools only reveal the workings of our external being in the realm of time and space.

However, there is an instrument through which we can know our true nature. This is the silent mind, that which is introverted and divested of all outer concerns. Once the mind reaches a state of deep calm and inner peace, disengaged from the distractions of the senses, it has the power to reflect the higher reality beyond all name and form.

## Self-Inquiry

The main approach of the yoga of knowledge is self-inquiry, directly looking into who we really are behind the veils of body and mind. It often begins with asking the question, "Who am I?"; not just at a mental or emotional level but with our full attention and energy. Through this question one learns to dive deep within, to the mind's origin located in the heart.

Yoga philosophy teaches us that there are three main aspects of our individual existence: our body, mind, and inner being. The physical body, with its limbs and organs, is the focus of our awareness, particularly when we take action in the external world. The mind is our psychological nature through reason, emotion, sensation, and other mental functions and activities. It is the inner focus of our awareness when we immerse ourselves in our thoughts, feelings, and memories. However, behind both body and mind dwells our inner being, an awareness of self and existence that is eternal, immutable, continuous, and content within itself. Yogic knowledge provides us with the direct understanding of our being beyond body and mind, name and form.

Have you ever had the sense that there is something in us that differs from the body and the mind? Deep inside of us is an essence of awareness that does not change through the processes of birth, growth, decay, and death. There is something in us that remains unperturbed and unshaken even when we are in great physical or emotional pain.

Note that we have a certain sense of self-identity that remains steady throughout our lives, despite changes in our jobs, beliefs, and bodies. We have a certain sense of being a whole person. Even if we happen to lose a limb, we don't want to be treated as less than a whole person. There is something within us that transcends death, which is why we seek immortality. That is our true self, Atman or Purusha, the goal of yoga and the place of unity with all.

If we trace the root of our thoughts, breath, or speech, we will find that they rise up out of a deeper sense of self or being in the heart—an inner core of profound knowing and deep feeling. Self-inquiry consists of questioning our shifting outer identity and coming to rest in the pure self, the "I am that I am" that does not depend upon any external reference, and which remains content in its own eternal peace, even without a body or mind.

This teaching of self-inquiry can be found in perhaps its clearest and most universal expression in the teachings of Ramana Maharshi, who is regarded as an enlightened sage of modern India. Traditionally it is found in the teachings of Shankara and the system of Advaita or nondualistic Vedanta.[41] But aspects of it permeate all the teachings of yoga.

# BHAKTI YOGA:

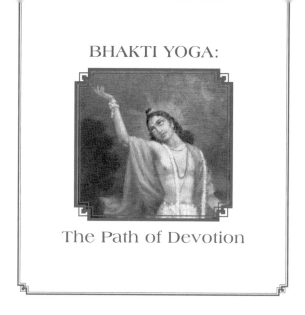

## The Path of Devotion

The vast literature of yoga reveals that the most common form of yoga practiced throughout the centuries in India has been Bhakti Yoga, the yoga of devotion. While there are only a few ancient texts on asanas, there are hundreds of tracts on devotion. The Bhakti Yoga Sutras of the sage Narada is a special text that addresses Bhakti Yoga in the same detail that the Yoga Sutras addresses the topic of Raja Yoga. Generally regarded as the highest of the yoga scriptures, the Bhagavad Gita of Sri Krishna also emphasizes Bhakti Yoga.

Like the yoga of knowledge, the yoga of devotion exists both as part of classical Raja Yoga and as a special yogic path of its own. It is also a key formulation of the Inner Yoga of meditation. Patanjali describes Ishvara pranidhana, devotion to the supreme divine being within us, as the quickest means to enter samadhi, the unitary state that is the goal of yoga.

Devotion rests upon surrender to the divine within one's deepest consciousness. This expression of surrender is called *namas* in Sanskrit. We find this term in many Sanskrit mantras to different deities, for example, "namah Shivaya." *Namaste* is a greeting that honors the divine presence in others.

Srimad Bhagavatam, one of the key texts on this subject, defines Bhakti Yoga according to nine factors:

1. **Shravana**: *listening to stories or teachings about God*
2. **Kirtana**: *singing the praises of God*
3. **Smarana**: *remembrance of God*
4. **Padasevana**: *service to God*
5. **Archana**: *worship of God*
6. **Vandana**: *praise of God*
7. **Dasya**: *becoming a servant of God*
8. **Sakhya**: *friendship with God*
9. **Atmanivedana**: *self-dedication or surrender to God*

Bhakti Yoga consists in concentrating one's mind, emotions, and senses on the divine, both externally and internally. This may involve temple worship, gatherings of devotees, service to the guru, and mantra and chanting in various forms. Its final stage of Atmanivedana is comparable to Ishvara pranidhana, surrender to the divine as one's inner self.

Bhakti Yoga often rests upon worshipping the divine in particular forms. These divine forms are called *devatas* in Sanskrit. They are not separate gods and goddesses, as polytheism, but rather a diverse approach to the infinite divine.

Yoga gives us the freedom to worship the divine in whatever form we like or as a formless entity. It follows the concept of *Ishta Devata*, or the "chosen deity." Yoga teaches us that we can worship the divine as father, mother, brother, sister, master, or beloved in human, animal, plant, or nature forms — however we like. After all, everything comes from God, and all things reveal to us some aspect of the universal reality. It is this inner freedom that is behind the many deities in the yoga tradition.

For those who may not want to use forms, one can also worship the divine as formless. Even so, one usually cultivates a relationship with the divine similar to that of father, mother, or beloved. We can worship the divine as truth, infinity, eternity, or other formless ways, but this usually takes us more in the direction of the yoga of knowledge.

The yoga of devotion teaches how to merge into the reality of divine love. As such, it is the sweetest of the yoga approaches and is often more easily accessible than the yoga of knowledge and formless approaches emphasizing the impersonal, the void, or emptiness. However, Bhakti Yoga has its elaborate philosophy as well. Many great devotional gurus have also been great thinkers and commentators, such as Ramanuja, Madhva, Chaitanya,[42] and Swami Narayan,[43] and have left many profound teachings for us to contemplate.

# Tantric and

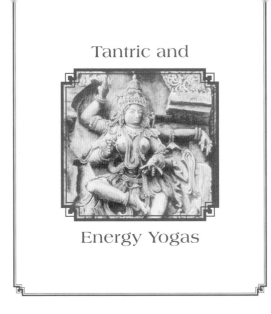

# Energy Yogas

Another aspect of inner yoga practices that has its special fascination, particularly in New Age circles, is working with the chakras and the energy of Kundalini, the internal power necessary to develop higher states of consciousness beyond the mind. Such energetic approaches to yoga usually employ pranayama along with mantra and meditation, as well as certain asanas and *mudras* (gestures), to stimulate the Kundalini to rise, which is necessary to open the chakras. These techniques are most commonly found in Tantric teachings.[44]

Kundalini is the secret evolutionary power of yoga hidden in the psyche that unfolds the deeper yogic processes within us. Great yogis worship the Kundalini as the power of the goddess or Shakti, which rules the entire universe. Kundalini is a higher energy of mind, prana, and speech. It is aroused by special mantras, pranayama, and meditative states of mind and heart.

In the yogic view, the chakras are centers of cosmic consciousness, not simply centers of physical or psychological energy. The yogi seeks to open the cosmic aspect of chakra energy to experience all of nature inside the self.

· Through opening the *root* or *earth* chakra (*Muladhara*), we come to experience all forms of the earth as part of our own deeper consciousness, being, and bliss.

· Through opening the *sex* or *water* chakra (*Svadhishthana*), we come to experience all forms of water and liquid in the universe as part of our own deeper lives.

· Through opening the *navel* or *fire* chakra (*Manipura*), we come to experience all forms of fire and light in the universe as part of our own greater light.

· Through opening the *heart* or *air* chakra (*Anahata*), we come to experience all forms of air and energy in the universe as part of our own greater breath.

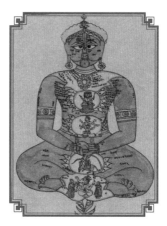

- Through opening the *throat* or *ether* chakra (*Vishuddha*), we come to experience all of space and the sound vibrations inherent within it.
- Through opening the *third eye* or *mind* chakra (*Ajna*), we come to experience all perceptual powers in the universe as aspects of our own greater vision.
- Through opening the *crown* or *lotus* chakra of the head (*Sahasrara*), we come to experience the divine consciousness, the higher self, reflected in our mind in a state of deep peace and profound bliss.



## Sexual Yoga Practices

Certain Tantric approaches use sacred sexuality as a yogic path. Despite the general identification of Tantra with sex in popular literature (much like that of yoga with asana), this aspect of Tantra is actually only a small portion of the Tantric system.[45]

Tantra teaches us how to turn our desires into forms of worship. If we do not succeed directly in the difficult task of transcending the body, we can at least turn all our bodily activities into sacred rituals. In this light, Tantra approaches sexuality as a ritual to be offered to the divine, the god and goddess within us. Such sacred sexuality is very different from mere hedonism. It requires dedication, a deep commitment to a partner, and an inward turning of the heart. Tantric texts outline the use of incense, aromas, flower offerings, mantra, and meditation as part of the process.

# Yoga, Tantra, and Magic ⚝

Yoga contains much of what can be called *occultism*, a study of the subtle worlds and their powers, including various forms of extrasensory perception. Yogis commonly achieve telepathy, subtle powers of seeing and hearing, the ability of astral travel, and the power to see the future.

In the Bhagavad Gita, Sanjaya relates the events of the battle occurring many miles away to King Dhritarashtra, using his divine vision born of the power of yoga. Ancient yoga texts such as the Yoga Vasishta speak of leaving body consciousness, visiting higher worlds, and even of time travel.

Such yogic powers make science fiction look mundane. After all, science fiction requires the use of technology. The yogi can travel through the entire universe without needing to leave the room where he or she sits. Developed yogic awareness makes it possible to move at will in the greater universe of consciousness.

However, there are lesser Tantrics who use occult powers to manipulate and control others, to gain worldly wealth or power, or even to harm people. This has very negative karmic consequences and should not be pursued. Yoga warns us against following such practices.

The deepest magic is the yogic union with the cosmic reality. If you are one in spirit with all, there is nothing external that you need to seek and no one outside yourself left to control. There is nothing in the universe that you need to seek, resist, or try to change. You are content and peaceful deep within, regardless of what happens in the world around you.

# Yoga as Mantra

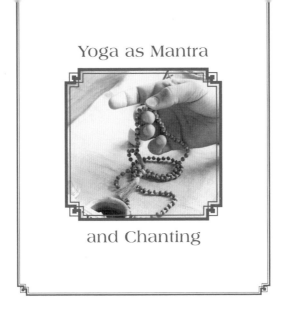

## and Chanting

Mantra plays a central role in all the branches of yoga, even where asana is not significant. In yoga approaches such as knowledge and devotion, where asana is secondary, mantra remains primary. Mantra is probably the most common tool of all yoga teachings. All yoga paths and teachings have their special mantras, sacred sounds, chants, and prayers that are the basis for all they do.

The chanting of mantras has remained an integral part of the Western yoga movement and has spawned its own set of music today in what is called the Kirtan movement. *Kirtan* is a Sanskrit word for chanting out loud or singing mantras, usually in a group setting, with the audience repeating the mantras that the main chanter sings. Even those who may not know the meaning of these chants often find the sound and the devotion inspired by them spiritually elevating.

In the Yoga Sutras, mantra is part of *svadhyaya, tapas,* and *Ishvara pranidhana,* the three main aspects of Kriya Yoga. Svadhyaya, or self-study, is often said to consist of the repetition of mantras. One of the main methods of tapas, or self-discipline, incorporates the use of mantras. And Ishvara pranidhana, or surrender to the divine, is mainly supported by the use of mantras, starting with OM or Pranava, the prime mantra indicating Ishvara.[46]

Mantras are special sacred sounds, songs, or even music. The classical literature of yoga and most of its mantras are in the Sanskrit language, which is called the "language of yoga" or the "language of the gods." Correct pronunciation and recitation of the mantras depends upon basic knowledge of Sanskrit. Mantras are of several types.

## Bija or Seed Mantras ✤

Bija or seed mantras are single-syllable mantras such as OM. Such primal sounds carry powerful forces that can heal the mind of unhealthy patterns, down to the subconscious level. They can be used to promote meditation[47] or applied as part of longer mantras for greater effectiveness. They can energize deities, chakras, and higher faculties.

### Important Bija Mantras

OM (om): for cosmic energy and higher awareness

AIM (aym): for the power of divine speech

HRIM (hreem): for opening the energy of the spiritual heart

KLIM (kleem): for promoting the energy of divine love

SHRIM (shreem): for increasing faith and devotion

KRIM (kreem): for developing the internal electrical
              energy of yoga

HUM (hoom): for the spiritual energy of fire
and discrimination

## Seed Sounds of the Five Elements

LAM: for the earth element and root chakra

VAM: for the water element and sex chakra

RAM: for the fire element and navel chakra

YAM: for the air element and heart chakra

HAM: for the ether element and throat chakra

(In all instances above, the "A" is pronounced like *e* in the English word *the*.)

# Divine Names ❀

Divine names are the names of the divine in its various
aspects, forms, and manifestations; for example, *Om
Namah Shivaya*, "OM reverence to Shiva." Such mantras usually
contain the name of the deity in the mantra. They may also
include other bija mantras or mantras using *namah*, meaning
"reverence to." There are many such name mantras that center
around a divine name.

Om Namo Bhagavate Vasudevaya
OM reverence to Bhagavan Vasudeva (Vishnu-Krishna)

Om Namo Narayanaya!
OM reverence to Narayana

Hare Krishna, Hare Rama
Mahamantra to Krishna

Kali Durge Namo Nama
reverence to the goddess as Kali and Durga

Similar name mantras occur in the Buddhist tradition with such reverence given to Buddha, Tara, Amitabha, or other Buddhist teachers.

## Extended Mantras ✼

Extended mantras are mantric statements, prayers, affirmations, and solicitations. They can be requests to the divine for grace, help, healing, or other assistance in life, whether for mundane or spiritual purposes. Or they can project certain teachings or truths.

Peace or *shanti* chants are prayers for universal welfare, peace, and happiness for all beings. Hymns of praise (*stotras*) are offered to various divine forms and teachers as an expression of devotion. Vedic chants (*suktas*) are extended mantras containing great powers of sound and meaning.

Important extended mantras include the Gayatri Mantra to the sun god for enlightening the mind and the Mahamrityunjaya Mantra to Lord Shiva for warding off suffering and calamity. Such mantras are too complex phonetically to provide here, and unfortunately tapes are not commonly available.

### Mantra in the Paths of Yoga

Bhakti Yoga rests upon chanting divine names. The yoga of knowledge has its special affirmations of higher truth called *Mahavakyas*, for example, Sarvam Khalvidam Brahma,[48] or "Everything is Brahman" (God or the absolute).

Kriya and Kundalini Yogas use special mantras along with pranayama and asana to awaken internal energies, including Kundalini and the chakras. Kundalini itself is said to consist of the essence of sound. Each chakra itself is a center, defined by certain sacred sounds.

# Usage of Mantras ✤

Mantras require long-term repetition, particularly with pranayama and meditation, for their full empowerment. Mantras can also be energized through holy places, powerful places in nature, and through such elements as fire and water. For spiritual mantras, it is best to receive the mantra from a guru or as part of a tradition. However, we can always feel free to chant the mantra of our Ishta Devata or the divine form that we personally choose to worship.

Mantras can also be used for mundane purposes. Mantras are used to promote healing in Ayurvedic medicine, particularly for psychological conditions, to counter negative planetary influences in Vedic astrology, and to harmonize the energies of one's dwelling in Vastu Shastra. Those adequately trained in these Vedic disciplines are taught such mantras and how to use them.

## The Mantra Yogi

A mantra yogi is one who follows the path of Mantra Yoga. In Mantra Yoga, the main focus is the mantra, which is a kind of asana for the mind. We repeat the mantra as a means of developing prana and awareness, and forget all else. The mantra connects us to the deity, our higher self, and the universal being, taking us through the vibrations of cosmic sound beyond space and time.

To be adept in Mantra Yoga is one of the greatest achievements of yoga practice. Consistently directing the mind, which is as changeable as the wind, is harder than controlling the body, which at least is fixed in form and structure. Mantras can change the patterns of our minds and prana, restructuring our life energies and expressions, and affording them higher levels of function.

PART 2: THE GREATER PRACTICES OF YOGA

If you want to benefit from yoga in its real depth, make some important mantras with your friends, and integrate them into your practice. Search out good teachers and gurus who can impart such mantras to you, even if you have to travel far or learn some Sanskrit.

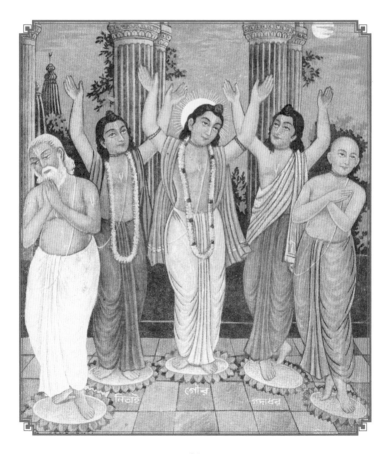

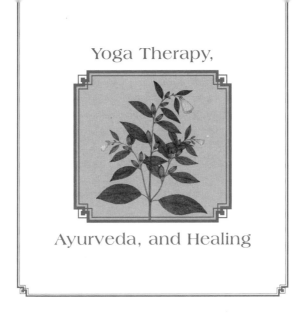

# Yoga Therapy, Ayurveda, and Healing

Most people initially come to yoga for physical healing, applying yoga postures to improve their health and energy, or to counter disease and injury. However, yoga is much more than just asanas for healing the body; it is part of a complete system of medicine for the body, mind, and spirit.

For healing purposes, traditionally yoga practices have been used according to the guidelines of Ayurveda, India's natural system of health and well-being. *Ayurveda*, which means the "science of life," is one of the world's oldest and most comprehensive healing systems. It has been practiced in India for thousands of years and today is spreading worldwide. In fact, where yoga has gone, Ayurveda is following in its footsteps, particularly as the yogic emphasis on healing and therapy continues to grow. The Ayurvedic aspect of yoga is bound to become one of the most important trends in yoga, as well as the most important aspect of yogic healing over time.[49]

Yoga and Ayurveda are sister sciences with Vedic roots in the older teachings of India. Yoga and Ayurveda share the same language of life and consciousness, viewing the universe and the human being through such shared factors as Purusha, prakriti, prana, and the five elements. Ayurveda adds an additional dimension through its profound explanation of how the body works: its view of the three *doshas*, or "biological humors," of *vata* (air), *pitta* (fire), and *kapha* (water). Ayurveda adapts diet, exercise, and lifestyle, including yoga practices, based upon the various mind-body types that arise through the doshas.

Whereas yoga indirectly addresses healing, Ayurveda approaches it as a primary focus, with a wealth of literature on physical and psychological disorders and detailed methods

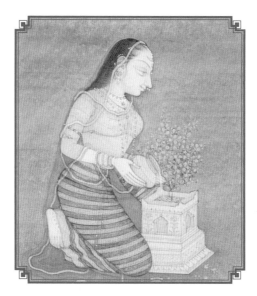

of diagnosis and treatment that include all aspects of yoga. Ayurveda provides us with a comprehensive yogic system of medicine, a full yogic medical care explaining diet, herbs, bodywork, and the application of yoga therapies from asana to meditation. Ayurveda addresses not only treatment but also disease prevention, including strengthening the immune system, rejuvenating the body, and promoting longevity.

Yoga is the Vedic system for dealing with spiritual suffering, the pain born of ignorance of our true nature, in which we forget the eternal welfare of our inner being for the outer pleasures of the body and mind. Ayurveda is the complementary Vedic system for addressing the diseases of body and mind. Ayurveda can be considered the medical branch of yoga. Ayurveda is yoga applied on a healing level, not just as a particular therapy but also as a complete system of right living and optimal well-being. *There is no separate traditional system of yogic medicine or yoga therapy apart from Ayurveda.* When traditional yoga has addressed health and disease, it has always done so through the language and methodology of Ayurveda. So if you want to really benefit from the healing powers of yoga, it is helpful to study Ayurveda along with it.

## Yoga Therapy and Ayurveda 🌿

Why is Ayurveda not commonly taught at yoga centers today? If Ayurveda is the medical system behind yoga, why haven't we heard more about it? There are particular reasons for this situation.

When yoga came to the Western world in the twentieth century, people naturally began viewing yoga according to the medical models predominant here. Alternative, and specifically Ayurvedic, models were not available in the West. Additionally, the British had closed all the Ayurvedic schools in India in the nineteenth century, which only began to reopen when the country gained its independence. So Ayurveda was not easy to learn in India either.

Having no access to Ayurveda, yoga teachers tried to adapt yoga practices, particularly yoga postures, according to the guidelines of modern medicine. Modern yoga therapy began to evolve from this basis, mainly in the use of yoga postures as an adjunct physical therapy for diseases as defined and treated by modern medicine. In this process, the yoga teacher prescribes yoga postures for patients based upon doctor or nurse recommendation and is not directly involved in treatment as a primary caregiver. While much benefit can derive from this approach, we cannot regard such a subordination of yoga to nonyogic systems of medicine as harnessing yoga's full healing potential.

Such a secondary application of yoga practices leaves the greater portion of yoga out of the picture, including pranayama, mantra, and meditation. It does not use the wisdom of yoga to address the internal medicine of diet and herbs either, but instead generally leaves the patient under the control of modern drug-oriented medicine. Yoga practices applied in this way lack the support of a yogic system of medicine as a whole. However, Ayurveda provides a full yogic and natural system of healing so that all yoga practices can have their full efficacy.

## Yoga and Psychology

Though many yoga practices, particularly asana and pranayama, provide health benefits for the body, classical yoga is primarily a method for healing the mind. The very definition of Patanjali's yoga as *chitta vritti nirodha*, or "calming the disturbances of the mind," aims at psychological and emotional healing. Therefore Ayurveda employs the classical yoga system of eight limbs as its main method of psychological healing. For any study of depth psychology, one should not forget the relevance of yoga and its understanding of consciousness from the subconscious to the highest awareness.

*Note:* We must provide a word of caution to the reader regarding applying yoga for any medical or healing purposes. Any medical treatment requires knowledge and expertise. Just as you cannot merely read a book on medicine and call yourself a doctor, similarly, real yoga therapy requires adequate training. While many yoga practices can be used for self-care, one must be careful in using these to treat acute diseases.

## Asana Therapy

Yoga asanas are the main external medicine of yoga. They work as a kind of self-massage to release tension and stress held in the bones, joints, and nerves. Yoga asanas are an important tool of physical healing, particularly for the musculoskeletal system and its problems, such as injuries or arthritis. Yet their benefits also extend through the circulatory system to the entire body, opening the channels for the flow of a deeper healing prana.

There is no disease that asana cannot help, even if it is only employed as a supplementary care method. Releasing blocked energy, asana can work wonders even for conditions that seem beyond its grasp. However, when a person has specific structural problems, an asana therapist must know how to adjust the exercise accordingly, as would any other good physical therapist.

We should note that practicing asanas incorrectly or excessively can cause serious injuries. The goal of asana therapy is not to force everyone to perform difficult postures but to facilitate easily moving and comfortably sitting in our particular type of body relative to our age and strength.

Asana should be balanced with the right diet.[50] Asana as exercise requires the right nutrition to support it. Yogic and Ayurvedic diets are important for all asana practitioners. They are vegetarian but of a nutritive nature, with whole grains, beans, root vegetables, seeds and nuts, and even dairy products. Unlike what some people might believe, a yogic diet does not require simply raw food, though such detox diets may be useful for short-term cleansing purposes.

## Prana Therapy ⚜

Pranayama is the main internal medicine of yoga. Breathing in more prana affords more healing energy for whatever we need. Its energizing effects are similar to taking herbs.

Pranayama works specifically on the respiratory and circulatory systems, the lungs and the heart, and their diseases. This includes colds, flu, allergies, lymphatic problems, and all manner of heart diseases. But pranayama can help with all health problems because prana underlies all the activities of the physical body and mind. And it does so in a much more direct way than asana, which works mainly from the outside.

Pranayama helps strengthen both the sensory and motor organs. It also increases the flow of blood and energy to the brain and nervous system, improving mental function. It can help counter psychological conditions such as depression or dullness. Deep belly breathing massages and stimulates the digestive tract as well, improving appetite, digestion, and elimination.

However, pranayama should be approached cautiously. One must be careful with strong pranayama practices—for example, very deep and rapid breathing—if one is suffering from heat, dehydration, low body weight, nervousness, or insomnia. Some health conditions are only treatable through proper nutrition and require special foods and herbs. Pranayama will not cure everything, but there is a great deal of adaptability in its possible applications, and there is little that some form of pranayama cannot help.

Pranayama is part of a greater system of pranic or energy healing. The yogi who has developed the healing power of prana can project it through touch or merely through his or her presence. Great yogis are natural pranic healers and bring with them the energy of the cosmic life wherever they go.

## Mantra and Meditation as Therapy

Mantra and meditation are the psychological medicines of yoga. Mantra helps us create a harmonious pattern of subtle sound vibration in our mental field, down to the subconscious level. This allows us to break deep-seated habits, patterns, and addictions, thereby removing the blockages, inhibitions, and residues of suffering and trauma. The right use of mantras can clear subconscious problems that psychoanalysis cannot remove.

Meditation puts the mind in a state of calm that allows the healing power of cosmic consciousness to enter into it. The still mind becomes a conduit for wisdom and love, which helps eliminate emotional and psychological problems. Meditation is the primary yoga therapy for relieving spiritual suffering. It affords us an inner bliss and happiness that nothing, not even death, can overcome.

### The Scope of Yoga Therapy

The scope of yoga therapy is vast, particularly if we include the many diagnostic procedures and healing tools of Ayurveda. Yoga therapy can help revolutionize both our physical and psychological systems of healing. With its integrative and naturalistic approach, such a yogic medicine provides the real basis for a planetary medicine. Yet yoga is not simply about personal healing; it aims to bring peace to the entire world, integrating humanity's different cultures into a greater unity that gives space for all to grow and flower according to their highest potential. Yoga's greatest healing gift is its ability to transport us beyond all suffering, by connecting us with the higher consciousness that is beyond birth and death, pleasure and pain, gain and loss.

## Conclusion: Entering the Universe of Yoga ✤

We have now completed a short but multifaceted introduction to the world of yoga. It has taken us from a popular exercise system for the body to an inner science for understanding mind and consciousness. Yoga is a gem with many facets, each a window to eternity and infinity. It allows us to cross all dimensions of life back to the origin of all existence. We are always on the great journey of yoga, whether we realize it or not.

A formal yoga practice allows us to consciously enter into the movement of transformation of our inner being. We all dwell in the universe of yoga, which is not just a part of what we do but the essence of who we are. Make yoga your own; discover the yoga within your deepest self as the basis of your unity with all.

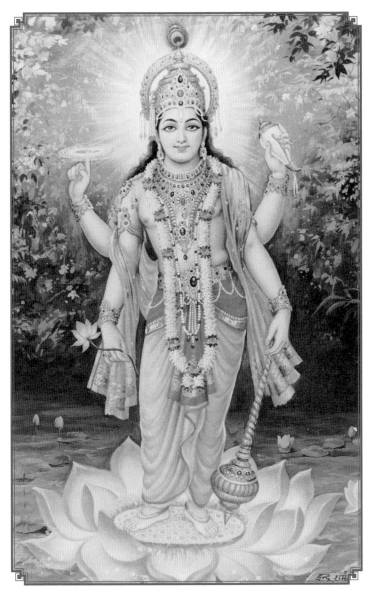

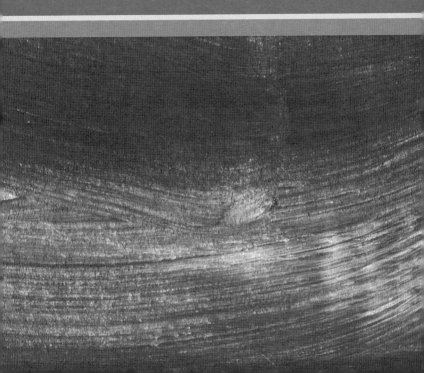

# APPENDIX AND RESOURCES

# Glossary of Terms ❧

**Abhyasa**: yoga practice

**Ahimsa**: nonharming

**Aparigraha**: nonpossessiveness

**Asana**: yoga postures

**Asteya**: nonstealing

**Atman**: higher self or inner being

**Ayurveda**: Vedic and yogic medicine

**Bhakti Yoga**: yoga of devotion

**Brahmacharya**: the proper use of sexual energy

**Brahman**: godhead or the absolute

**Buddhi**: higher mind

**Chikitsa**: therapy

**Chitta**: mind in the broadest sense

**Devi**: goddess

**Dharana**: concentration

**Dharma**: universal law

**Dhyana**: meditation

**Hatha Yoga**: yoga of technique

**Ishvara**: God as the cosmic lord

**Ishvara pranidhana**: surrender to the divine

**Jnana Yoga**: yoga of spiritual knowledge

**Kaivalya**: realization of the Purusha

**Karma**: service, action

**Kriya**: action or technique

**Laya**: mergence

**Mantra**: primal sound

**Moksha**: freedom, liberation

Nirodha: control, concentration

Niyama: yogic lifestyle practices

Prakriti: nature

Prana: vital energy

Pranayama: development or control of prana

Pratyahara: internalization of mind and prana

Purusha: higher self or inner being

Samadhi: deep inner absorption

Samyama: deep yogic concentration

Santosha: inner contentment

Satya: truthfulness

Saucha: purity

Shakti: cosmic power or goddess

Svadhyaya: self-study

Tantra: energetic yoga teachings

Tapas: striving, aspiration, internal heat

Vairagya: nonattachment

Vichara: examination

Viveka: inner discrimination

Yajna: sacrifice

Yama: yogic observances

## End Notes ❀

[1] Yoga Sutras I.2 and I.3.

[2] Bhagavad Gita II.48.

[3] Bhagavad Gita II.50.

[4] Bhagavad Gita VI.23.

[5] Katha Upanishad VI.11.

[6] Katha Upanishad VI.11.

[7] Svestasvatara Upanishad I.3, Dhyana Yoga.

[8] Katha Upanishad II.12, Adhyatma Yoga.

[9] Exercise is called *vyayama* in Sanskrit. The term does not occur in the Yoga Sutras. A healing therapy is called *Chikitsa* in Sanskrit. While there are many Chikitsa texts, these basically belong to Ayurvedic medicine. Yoga Chikitsa very rarely occurs as a term, and texts of this nature are very hard to find. It does not occur in the Yoga Sutras either.

[10] Similar to its classification of different types of samadhi.

[11] For example, the three-headed form of Shiva sitting in meditation posture as the lord of the animals can be found in Harappan seals dated from 2700 BCE in India, just as it can be found in Indian art today.

[12] We find the heart emphasized in traditional teachings from the ancient Upanishads to the modern teachings of the great enlightened sage, Ramana Maharshi.

[13] This is known as the *guru-shishya-parampara* in Sanskrit.

[14] Yoga Darshana forms a pair with the Samkhya system, which enumerates the main principles (*tattvas*) of cosmic existence starting with Purusha and prakriti, or spirit and matter. The main classical text on Samkhya is the Samkhya Karika of Ishvara Krishna (not Krishna of the Gita) from around 400 AD, though Samkhya, like Yoga, is based on much older teachings. It is often studied along with the Yoga Sutras.

[15] For example, the Hatha Yoga Pradipika IV.3–4 identifies Raja Yoga and Samadhi with Advaita or nonduality, whereas the Samkhya system that Patanjali follows is usually regarded as dualistic.

[16] Mahabharata, Shanti Parva, Moksha Dharma Parva 350.65. Also the Brihad Yogi Yajnavalkya Smriti 12.5.

[17] Rig Veda X.121, Hiranyagarbha Sukta.

[18] One could argue that the older Hiranyagarbha tradition of yoga, as taught in the Bhagavad Gita and the Mahabharata, and rooted in the Vedas, is the real tradition of yoga, of which the Yoga Sutra tradition of Patanjali is just one expression.

[19] Yoga Sutras, I.26 deems Ishvara the ultimate guru.

[20] Bhagavad Gita IV. 1–3.

[21] Bhagavad Gita IV. 5–8.

[22] Mahabharata, Ashvamedhika Parva, Anu Gita, XIX.15, for example, mentions teaching the unequaled Yoga Shastra.

[23] The Aitareya Upanishad III specifically teaches the process of self-inquiry.

[24] It is said to relate the complete teaching of yoga, yoga *vidhim ca krtsnam*, Katha Upanishad VI.18.

[25] Particularly Svetashavatara II.

[26] Matsya Purana I.13. 17–19.

[27] Rig Veda II.62.10.

[28] Rig Veda VII.59.12.

[29] Rig Veda IV.40.5.

[30] Refer to the Bhagavad Gita IV for different types of yoga practices, such as pranayama as yajnas.

[31] Like the Yoga Vasishta or Adhtyatma Ramayana.

[32] For example, Vasishta Samhita V deals with how the breath relates to the planets and signs of the zodiac at different times of the day.

[33] Hatha Yoga Pradipika I.1; Shiva as Adi Nath, the primal guru of Hatha Yoga.

[34] Not to be confused with Ashtanga Yoga as a modern asana style.

[35] For example, the Vasistha Samhita, another ancient yoga text apart from Patanjali, emphasizes yoga of the eight limbs. So do many others. See Vasistha Samhita I.31.

[36] Yoga Sutras I.12–13.

[37] The fruit of Svadhyaya in the Yoga Sutras II.44 is considered the vision of the Ishta Devata or one's chosen form of the divine for worship.

[38] Yoga Sutras II.1.

[39] Many Tantric Yoga texts address this topic.

[40] Yoga Sutras III.4.

[41] As in Shankara's text, Vivekachudamani, the Crest Jewel of Discrimination.

[42] Chaitanya is often regarded as an incarnation of Krishna himself.

[43] An important teacher from eighteenth-century Gujarat.

[44] Though not recent, Arthur Avalon and Sir John Woodroofe's books on Tantra are among the best, as are Jaidev Singh's work on Kashmiri Shaivism.

[45] Also, much of modern popular Tantra is based on modern psychology, for example, the work of Wilhelm Reich.

[46] Yoga Sutras I.27–28.

[47] The Transcendental Meditation movement does this, as does the primal-sound therapy of Dr. Deepak Chopra.

[48] Chandogya Upanishad III.14.1.

[49] For example, Swami Ramdev, probably the most popular yoga teacher and yoga therapist in India today, emphasizes Ayurveda and its connection to yoga.

[50] For example, the Hatha Yoga Pradipika mentions this.

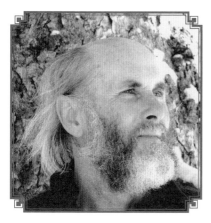

## About the Author ❀

D r. David Frawley (Pandit Vamadeva Shastri) is the
author of more than twenty books on the greater yoga
tradition, covering Ayurveda, Vedic astrology, Vedanta, and
the Vedas themselves. His books have been published in
more than a dozen languages and are commonly considered
as authoritative texts in their respective fields. In India he is
regarded as perhaps the most well-known Western exponent of
traditional Vedic knowledge.

Frawley is the director of the American Institute of Vedic
Studies in Santa Fe, New Mexico, and helps run Vedic
schools and training programs in North America, South
America, Europe, and India. More information on his
work can be found at his website (www.vedanet.com), which
contains a variety of resources in all the Vedic fields for
students to draw upon.

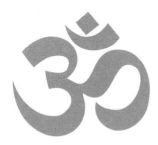

## Wisdom Series

The main text was typeset in MrsEaves.
The sidebars and main header text was
typeset using Berthold Akzidenz Grotesk.

All Mandala Wisdom Library books
are printed on 100gsm matte art text,
with endpapers printed on 120gsm
woodfree paper.

Series Editor
Arjuna van der Kooij

Designer
Mary Teruel